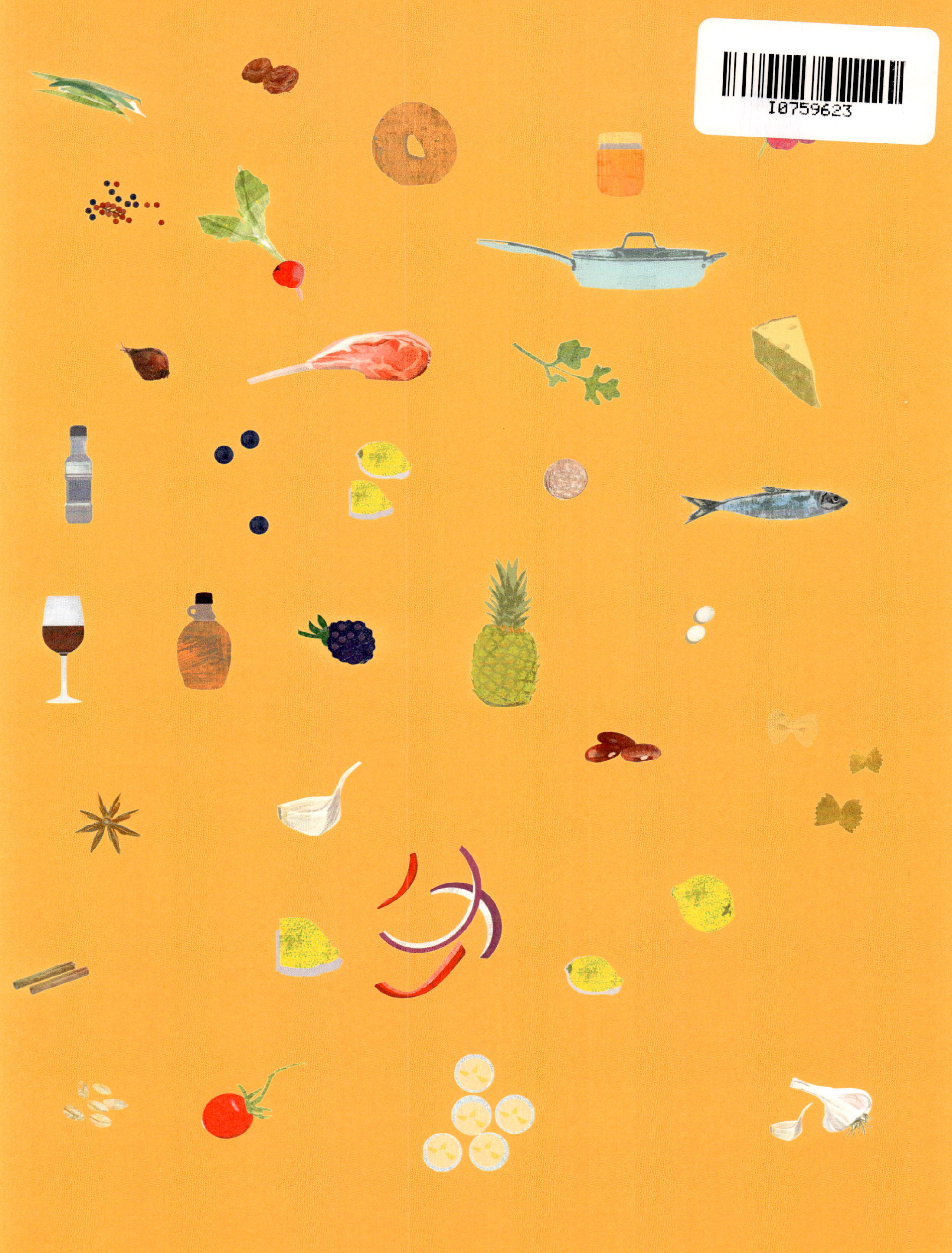
I0759623

Cook Improv: Fresh Foundations

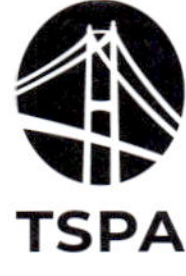

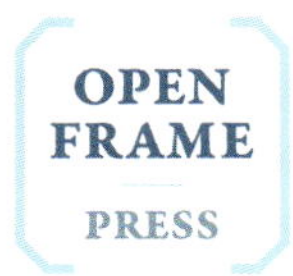

Tucker Herbert
CookImprov: Fresh Foundations

Published by Open Frame Press

First Edition

Illustration | Lou Baker Smith
Art Direction | Kat Catmur
Graphic Design | Karen Constanti
Editor | Judith Doyle
Author Portrait Photography | Hoon Bae
Cover Design | Kat Catmur
Cover Illustration | Lou Baker Smith
Publishing Management | TSPA The Self Publishing Agency, Inc.
theselfpublishingagency.com

ISBN: 979-8-9987902-0-1

cookimprov.com

Library of Congress Cataloging-in-Publication Data
Herbert, Tucker, author. | Baker Smith, Lou, illustrator.
CookImprov: Fresh Foundations/Tucker Herbert;
illustrations by Lou Baker Smith.
Subjects: LCSH: Cooking. | LCGFT: Cookbooks.
Library of Congress Control Number: 2025913704
Los Angeles, California

Cook Improv: Fresh Foundations

Frameworks for Inspired Breakfast, Brunch, Lunch, and Meal Prep

Tucker Herbert

Unlock your creativity, eat healthier, and cook with whatever you have on hand.

Contents

Frameworks roughly organized from "foundational" to more complex.

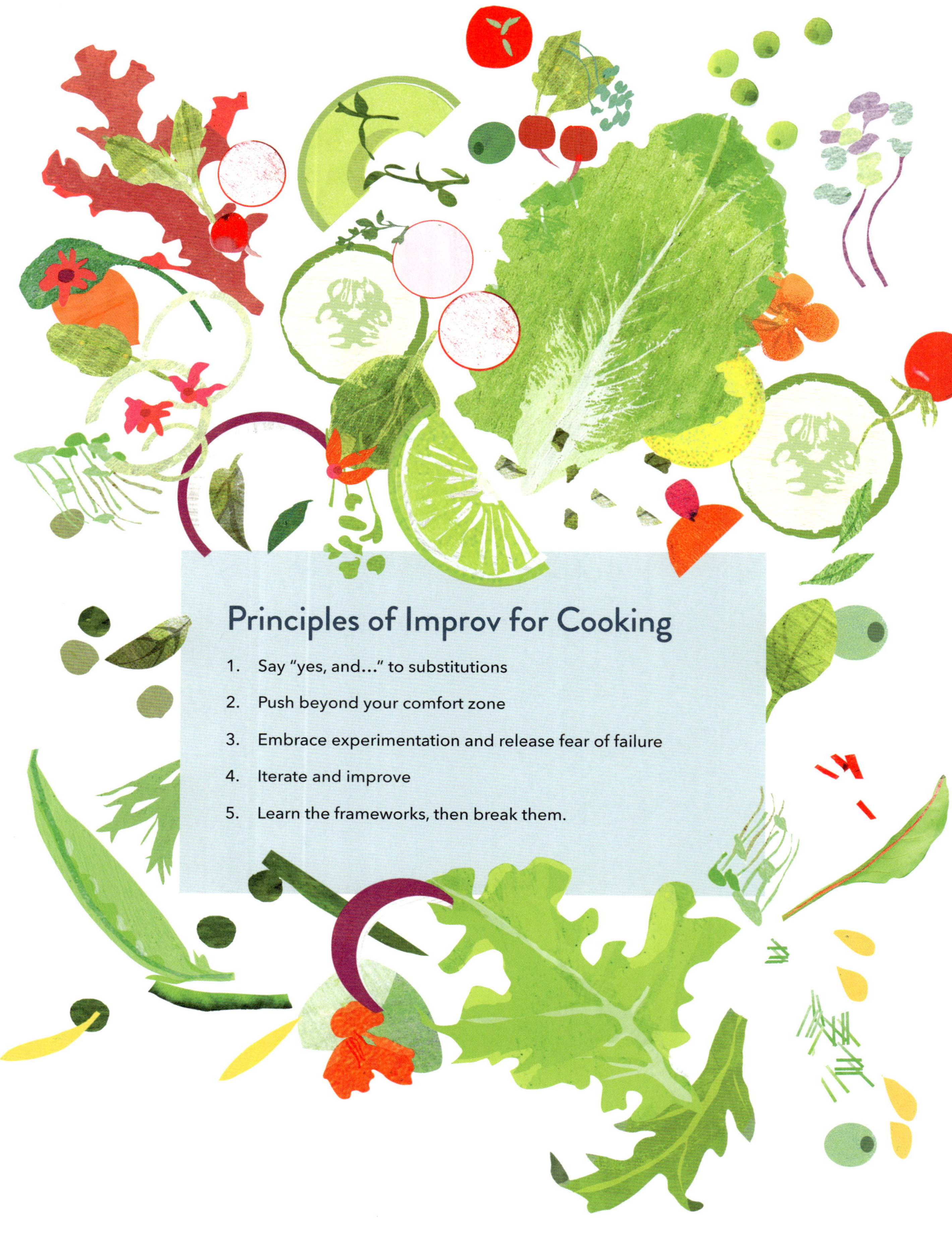

Principles of Improv for Cooking

1. Say "yes, and..." to substitutions
2. Push beyond your comfort zone
3. Embrace experimentation and release fear of failure
4. Iterate and improve
5. Learn the frameworks, then break them.

Consider this your catalyst to become a bold improvisational cook. Where cookbooks give you rules, here you'll find the tools to innovate. Start by learning the initial frameworks, practicing until you're comfortable creating your own variations.

Once mastered, these frameworks serve as a quick reference for proportions and ingredient inspiration.

The improv approach minimizes ingredient purchases by relying on kitchen staples and flexible substitutions – freeing you to grab whatever catches your eye at the farmer's market, knowing you can incorporate any fruit, vegetable, or protein into a variety of dishes.

It all starts with the salad.

Master the salad, and the frameworks that follow will flow more naturally, as you build foundational skills to invent entirely new dishes.

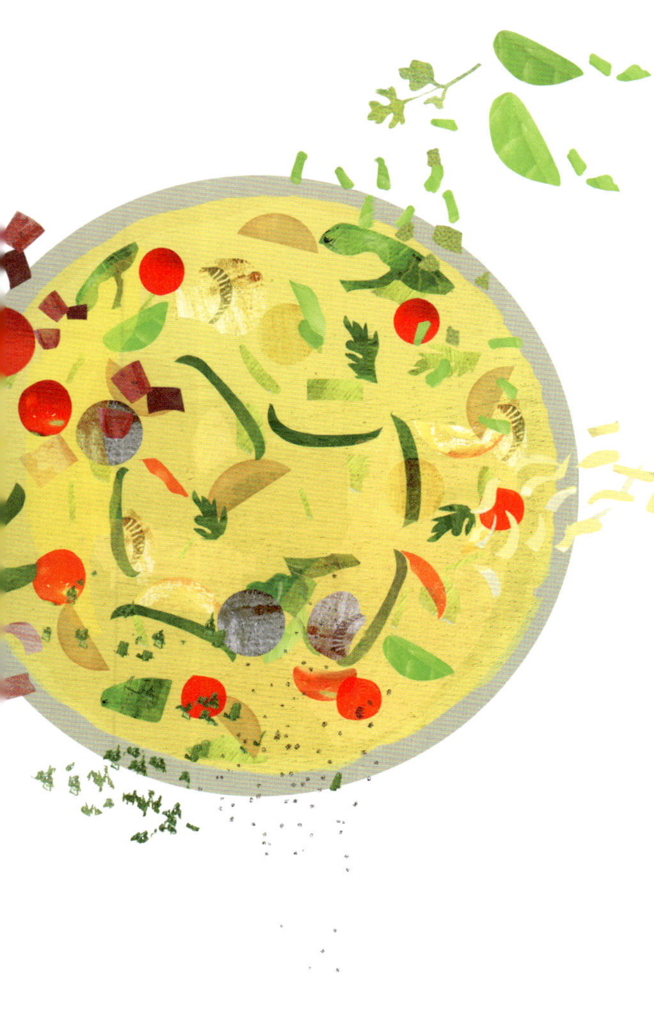

How to Use this Book

- Each dish has a Framework as well as Tips and Example Pairings - use the Framework as your primary guide
- Remember to season to taste with salt and pepper (this generally is not called out)
- If the suggested quantity for an ingredient starts at 0, it's optional
- Garnish suggestions are always optional
- Categories and Ingredients are typically capitalized (and often underlined) in frameworks to guide the eye and ease improvisation - elsewhere, they may appear in lowercase - it's all about clarity
- Trust your judgment and adapt recipes to suit your preferences and ingredients on hand

Example Pairings

- Think of these as "training wheels" if you're wondering where to start from an improvisational perspective
- Ingredients from the same category are listed either to indicate sequence (when timing is important) or in order of suggested quantities
- Ingredients considered foundational in the framework may not be listed here

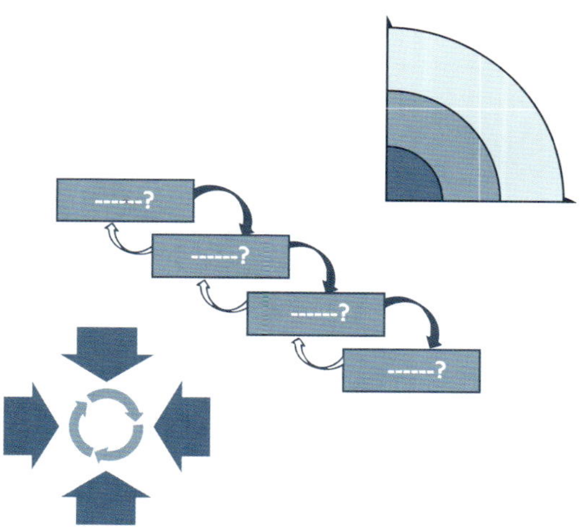

Frameworks

The much-decried tools (or shackles) of MBAs and consultants alike, to optimize, prioritize, rationalize and strategize - they can also liberate. If you love frameworks, this is your book; if you'd like to love them, this is your cupid. Free yourself with these frameworks to break from the constraints of prescriptive recipes.

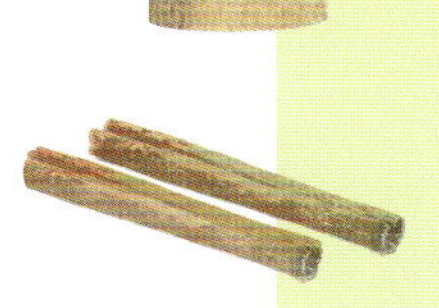

Skills You Will Develop through CookImprov

1. Build intuition for pairings
2. Develop a sense for balancing proportions
3. Season to taste by cycling through:
    - Does it need more salt?
    - Does it need more pepper?
    - Would more spice/sweetness enhance it?
    - Could a touch of citrus brighten it up?

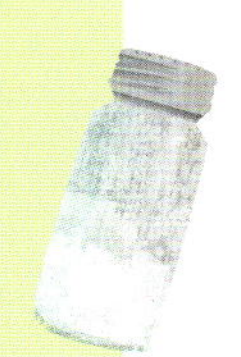

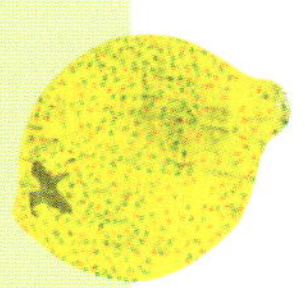

Key

- CookImprov favorite creations
- CookImprov take on classic dishes
- Vegetarian
- Vegan
- Comfort Foods
  Most CI dishes are health-forward, these are for times you're looking to indulge

Measurements

1t	1 Teaspoon	5 mL
1T	1 Tablespoon	15 mL
1 lb	1 Pound	450 g
1 oz *(weight)*	Ounce	~30 g
1 oz *(liquid)*	Fluid Ounce	~30 mL
1c	1 Cup	240 mL
1″	1 inch	~2 cm

Conversions rounded to simplify scaling.

It all starts with mastering the salad...

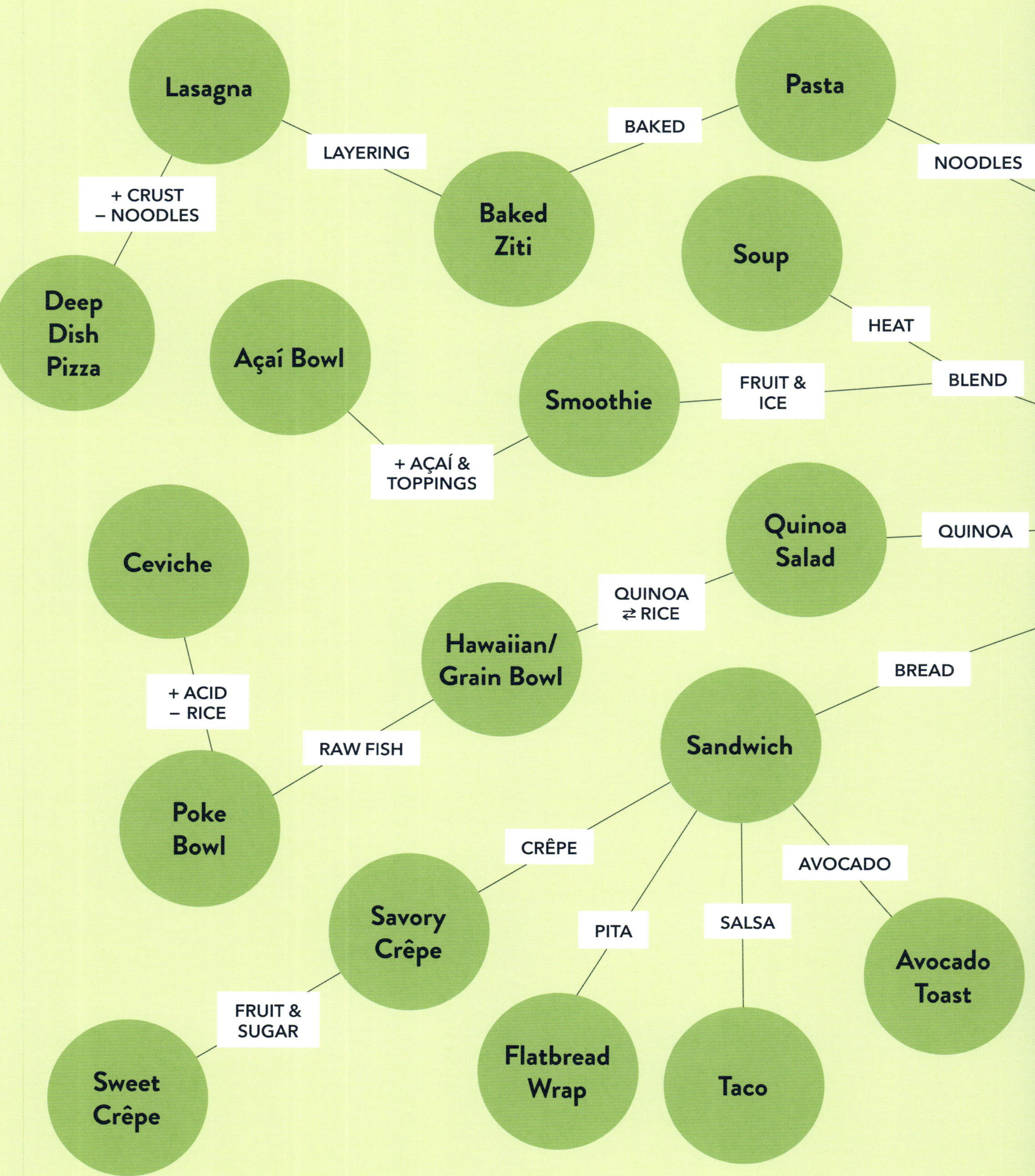

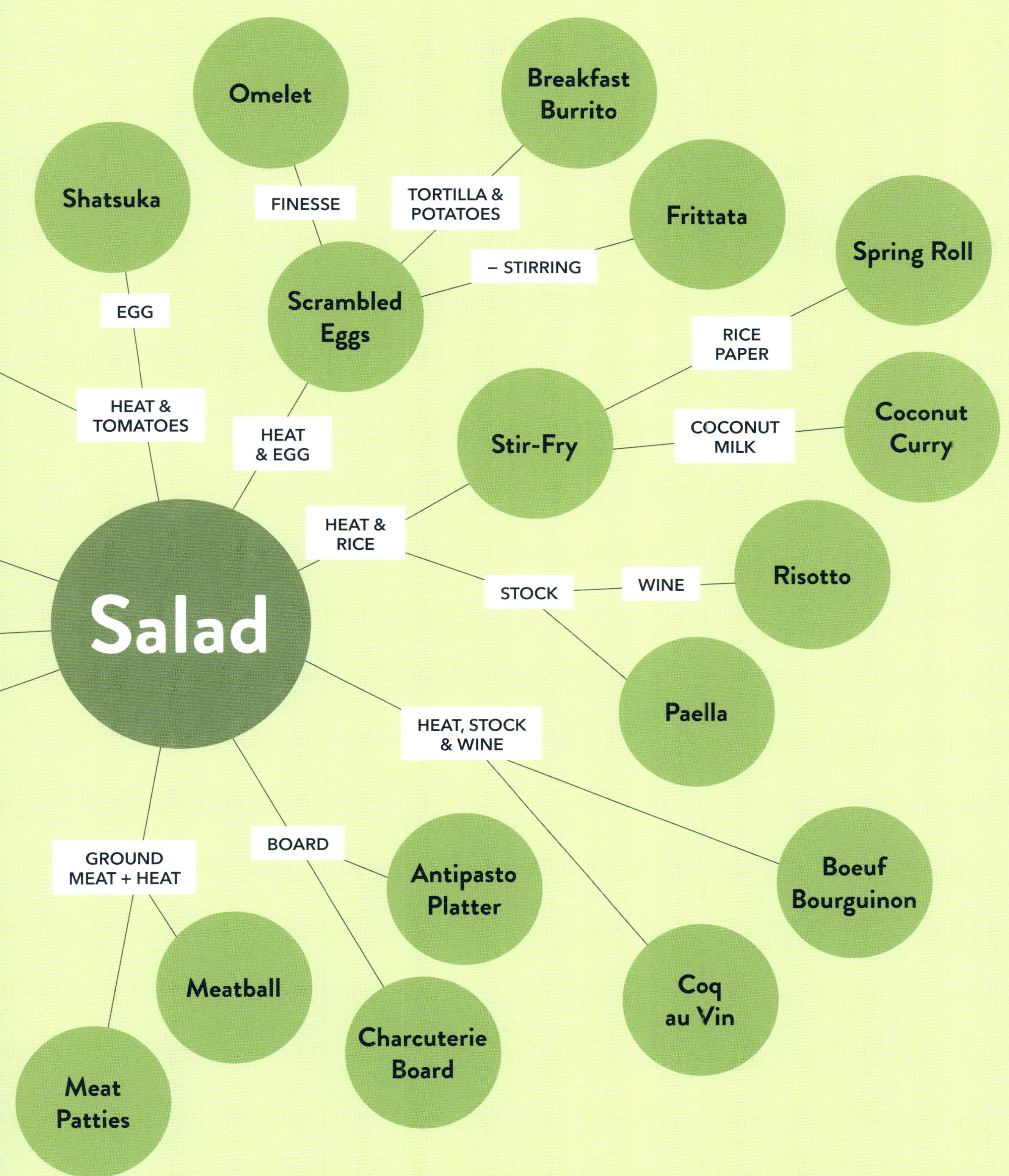

...and then realizing how fundamentally similar other dishes are.

Introducing the Salad Framework

Salad Categories

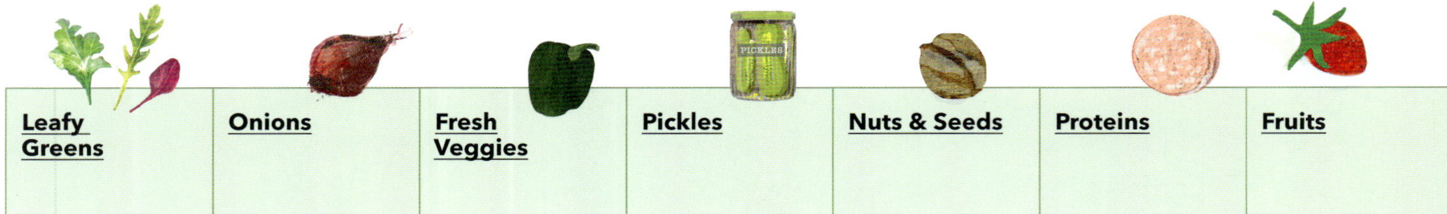

Flip page to unveil the complete Salad Framework

Shift from thinking about specific ingredients to an expanded view of ingredient categories.

Find key steps distilled to their most foundational parts with explanations on how to handle each category's ingredients.

What is a Salad?

We know a salad when we see one, yet what defines it?

Salads can range from lightly dressed greens to mixtures featuring fruits, meats, cheeses, pickles, and nuts. So, what is the common thread?

Think of a salad as a flexible combination of ingredients from key categories balanced to complement each other. This perspective reveals how other dishes can also be deconstructed and recomposed.

Everything, in essence, is a salad.

Unleash your abilities for culinary invention, discovering how to create delicious, adaptable meals – and have a blast doing it.

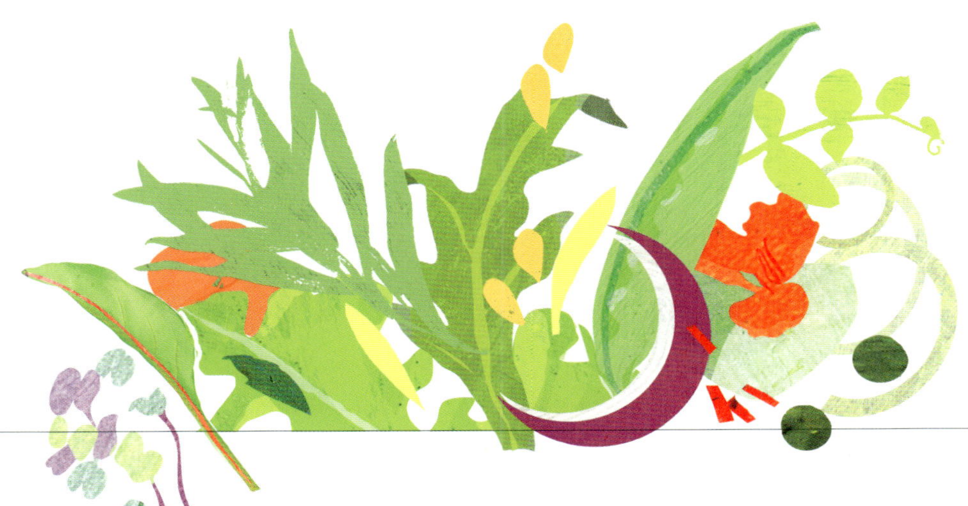

Ultimate Salad Framework

Whether tossing ingredients together or crafting something memorable, let this framework inspire confidence and creativity.

Start by thinking of your salad base as leafy greens with olive oil, lemon juice, salt and pepper. Then build texture, contrast, and flavor by selecting ingredients across categories.

Salad Base

Combine desired ingredients in bowl

Leafy Greens *1/4 – 1/2 head lettuce*	**Onions** *1/4 onion if sautéed, less otherwise*	**Fresh Veggies** *may include multiple*	**Pickles** *reduce oil/acid, salt in dressing to balance*	**Nuts & Seeds** *optional; toasted, crushed*	**Proteins** *optional; chopped*	**Fruits** *include selectively*
• Butter Lettuce • Romaine • Endive • Leafy Green Mix • Baby Arugula • Baby Spinach	• Shallot • Red Onion • Yellow Onion • Green Onion *Consider sautéing with olive oil & garlic*	• Bell Pepper • Tomato • Avocado • Cucumber • Mushroom (Garlic-sautéed) • Carrot • Broccoli	• Artichoke • Sun-dried Tomato • Pimiento • Banana Pepper • Olive • Carrot • Beet • Heart of Palm	• Pistachio • Cashew • Almond • Pine Nut • Peanut • Macadamia • Walnut, Pecan • Sunflower Seed	• Chicken - roasted/ sautéed • Cured Meat • Bacon • Egg • Shrimp • Smoked Salmon • Canned Fish	• Pear • Pomegranate • Fig • Apricot • Tangerine • Peach • Apple • Grapefruit

Dressing

Mix together; pour over salad just before serving

Oil *1-2t*	**Acid** *1/4 lemon or 1-2t*	**Salt & Pepper** *a pinch/to taste*	**Cheeses** *optional; grated/crumbled*	**Herbs** *optional; fresh or dried*	**Seasonings** *include selectively*
• Olive • Avocado • Toasted Sesame • Peanut • Chili • Truffle	• Lemon Juice • Red Wine/Sherry Vinegar • Balsamic Vinegar • Lime Juice • Rice Vinegar • Orange Juice	• Sea Salt • Kosher Salt • Himalayan Salt • Mixed Peppercorn • Black Pepper • White Pepper • Togarashi	• Parmesan • Feta • Mozzarella • Burrata • Manchego • Cheddar • Blue	• Herbes de Provence • Basil • Oregano • Tarragon • Rosemary • Thyme • Mint • Cilantro • Parsley	• Dijon, Whole Grain or Honey Mustard* • Ponzu/Soy Sauce* • Ginger • Five-Spice • Coriander, Cumin • Cardamom ** If using, reduce Acid and Salt for balance.*

Suggested quantities are per person.

Ingredients flow left to right from essential to optional, and top to bottom from easiest to pair to those needing more consideration.

Tips on how to apply

Getting Started

You likely have most of the foundational ingredients already: olive oil, vinegar, salt, pepper, an onion, and perhaps some parmesan - so the only thing you need to grab is lettuce.

- Level up: Stock long shelf life additions like jarred artichokes, banana peppers, roasted pistachios, cashews, dried figs, or apricots to quickly elevate your salad game.

Keeping it Healthy

Err on the side of less dressing - you can always add more.

Pairings & Balance

While most of these ingredients pair well together, ingredients lower on each list (e.g., canned fish, blue cheese, soy sauce) require consideration on how to pair.

- Regional Inspiration: Let global flavors (e.g., France, Italy, East Asia) guide combinations.
- Calibration: Adjust dressing based on ingredients - if adding sun-dried tomatoes in oil, pickled vegetables, or salted nuts, reduce the oil, acid, or salt in dressing to maintain balance.

Other Tips

- Proportions: Strong flavors like pickles, dried fruit, and nuts go a long way - start small.
- Chopping: Make everything bite-sized so no knife is needed while eating.
- Spin: Use a salad spinner to keep leafy greens crisp.
- Assembly: Apply dressing directly to greens, as they need it most (this also enables you to use less dressing overall).
- Dressing Base: View olive oil as your go-to base, then choose balsamic, sherry vinegar, or lemon juice.
- Experiment Freely: These ingredients are just a starting point - mix, match, and create - you're the master chef!

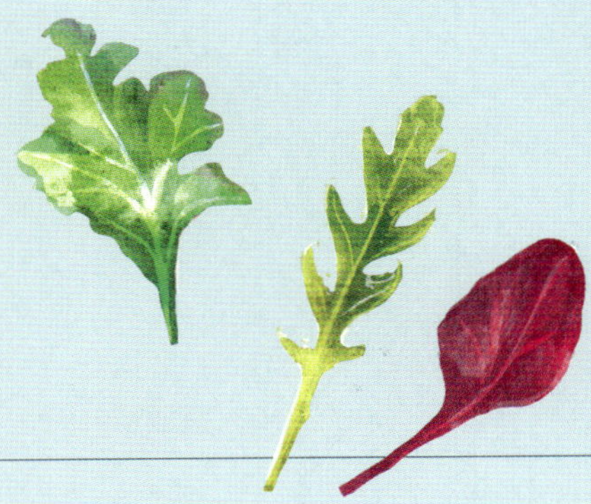

Example pairings

CookImprov Classic

Butter Lettuce, Sautéed Red Onion, Bell Pepper, Sun-dried Tomato, Pistachio, Parmesan

Dressing: Olive Oil, Lemon Juice, Salt, Pepper

Tangerine Chicken Macadamia

Leafy Green Mix, Green Onion, Cucumber, Tangerine, Roasted Chicken, Macadamia Nut

Dressing: Sesame Oil, Ponzu Sauce, Pepper

Romaine Artichoke Parmesan

Romaine Lettuce, Thinly Sliced Shallot, Cherry Tomato, Marinated Artichoke Heart, Parmesan

Dressing: Olive Oil, Lime Juice, Salt, Pepper

Arugula Avocado Cashew

Baby Arugula, Sautéed Shallot, Avocado, Cashew

Dressing: Olive Oil, Lemon Juice, Salt, Pepper, Herbes de Provence

Caramelized Onion, Mushroom & Fig

Leafy Green Mix, Caramelized Onion, Sautéed Cremini Mushroom, Walnut, Dried Fig

Dressing: Olive Oil, Sherry Vinegar, Salt, Pepper

Dijon Frisée Banana Pepper & Pepperoni

Frisée Lettuce, Thinly Sliced Shallot, Cucumber, Marinated Banana Pepper, Chopped Pepperoni

Dressing: Olive Oil, Dijon Mustard, Salt, Pepper, Tarragon

Fruit Salad Framework

Shine the spotlight on fruit for freshness, flair, and unexpected depth.

Fruit salad is tragically underrated – done right, it's as close as dessert gets to tasting like a sunrise and feeling like a vitamin. Start by mixing fruits across categories to hit contrast in flavor, texture, and color. Then break the rules: while fruit's the star, a handful of nuts, a crumble of soft cheese, or a sliver of onion or cured meat can add unexpected complexity.

Salad Base

Combine desired ingredients in bowl

Tree/Stone Fruits *sliced*	**Berries & Melon** *bite-sized*	**Tropical & Citrus** *peeled, sliced*	**Other Fruits** *bite-sized*	**Cheeses** *optional; grated/crumbled*	**Veggies** *optional; sliced*	**Onion & Meat** *include selectively; very thinly sliced*
• Peach • Pear • Apple • Plum • Apricot • Dates	• Strawberry • Blackberry • Blueberry • Raspberry --- • Honeydew • Cantaloupe • Watermelon • Galia	• Mango • Pineapple • Banana • Kiwi --- • Orange • Grapefruit • Kumquat – whole or sliced	• Grapes • Pomegranate • Fig • Guava • Coconut – shredded • Rambutan • Lychee • Persimmon	• Burrata • Mozzarella • Mascarpone • Goat • Feta • Blue	• Avocado • Cucumber • Cherry Tomato • Heart of Palm • Artichoke • Arugula	• Red Onion • Shallot • Sweet Onion • Green Onion --- • Prosciutto • Spanish Chorizo • Other Cured Meats

Dressing

Mix together; pour over salad just before serving

Acid *recommended*	**Fresh Herbs** *optional; chopped*	**Oil** *optional, 0–1t*	**Sweet** *if desired*	**Nuts** *include selectively; toasted or candied*	**Seasonings** *include selectively and sparingly*	**Yogurt** *include selectively*
• Lemon Juice • Lime Juice • Grapefruit Juice • Orange Juice • Red Wine/Sherry Vinegar • Balsamic Vinegar – reduced	• Basil • Mint • Cilantro • Tarragon • Lavender • Shiso	• Olive • Avocado • Sesame • Chili	• Honey • Simple Syrup • Maple Syrup • Chocolate – shaved	• Cashew • Almond • Macadamia • Walnut • Pecan • Pistachio	• Salt • Pepper • Chili – thinly sliced • Cayenne/Paprika/ Tajín • Ginger • Cardamom • Cinnamon/Clove	Greek or Traditional: • Plain • Vanilla • Fruit-flavored • Chocolate

Suggested quantities are per person.

Ingredients flow left to right from essential to optional, and top to bottom from easiest to pair to those needing more consideration.

Tips on how to apply

Getting Started

Having citrus and fresh herbs on hand helps elevate fruit salads – beyond that, it's all about what you have or what looks best at the market.

Keeping it Healthy

Fruits are packed with nutrients and natural sugars, making them a great option in moderation. Keep portions in check or serve as a nutritious dessert – far healthier than refined-sugar-heavy baked goods or ice cream.

Pairings & Balance

Use what you love, and you won't go wrong here. Contrast tart and sweet fruits, balance juicy with crisp textures, and consider herbs, spices, or citrus to add depth.

- Dressing: Flip the classic vinaigrette on its head with a citrus-forward base, just enough oil to carry it, some herbs, and perhaps a whisper of honey.

Other Tips

- Citrus: Peel most citrus (other than kumquats), and then either break into slices or cross-cut discs – either way, remove as much membrane as possible.
- Dried Fruit: Use sparingly – it may disrupt the balance of fresh, juicy textures.

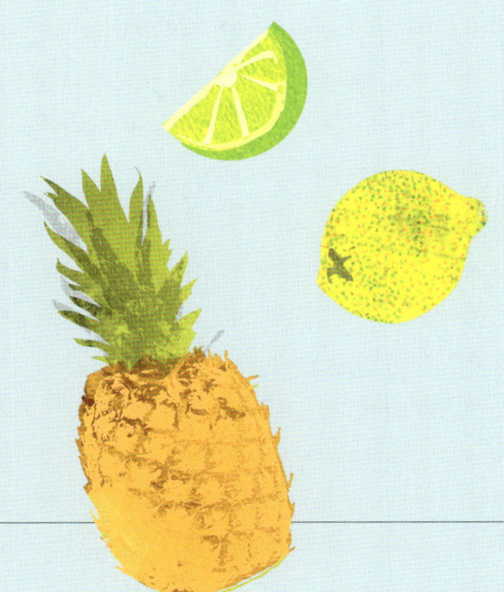

Example pairings

Honeydew Berry

Honeydew Melon, Blackberry, Strawberry; optional: Ricotta

Dressing: Lemon Juice, Tarragon, Honey, Salt

Melon Prosciutto

Peach, Avocado, Shallot, Pecan; optional: Arugula, Burrata

Dressing: Balsamic, Lemon Juice, Olive Oil, Honey, Basil

Moroccan Orange

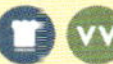

Blood Orange, Red Onion, Pistachio; optional: Black Olive

Dressing: Lime, Olive Oil, Paprika, Salt, Pepper, Mint

Modified Waldorf

Apple, Grape, Candied Walnut; optional: Lettuce, Celery, Dried Date, Goat Cheese

Dressing: Plain Greek Yogurt, Lemon Juice, Salt

Watermelon Cucumber Feta

Watermelon, Cucumber, Feta, optional: Red Onion, Arugula

Dressing: Lime/Lemon Juice, Olive Oil, Salt, Mint; optional: Black Pepper

Peach Avocado Pecan

Peach, Avocado, Shallot, Pecan; optional: Arugula, Burrata

Dressing: Balsamic, Lemon Juice, Olive Oil, Honey, Basil

Tropical

Mango, Pineapple, Banana, Shredded Coconut

Dressing: Lime Juice, Salt (just a pinch)

Quinoa Salad Framework

Turn quinoa into a hearty, flavorful base - perfect for layering texture, contrast, and nutrition.

This framework parallels the Ultimate Salad, with quinoa as your foundational ingredient. Dress quinoa directly to enhance flavor, then build across multiple categories.

Salad Base

Prepare and chill Quinoa; combine desired ingredients in bowl

Quinoa *0.75c dry; rinsed, boiled, chilled*	**Veggies** *2-4 types; chopped*	**Onions** *1 small; diced*	**Cheeses** *2-6 oz; cubed*	**Legumes** *1-2 types; steamed, chilled*	**Pickles/Leafy Greens** *0-2 types; chopped*	**Seeds & Nuts** *optional; toasted*
• White • Rainbow/Tri-Color • Red • Black	• Tomato • Bell Pepper • Corn - steamed • Avocado • Cucumber • Carrot - shredded • Pea, Snow Pea - blanched	• Red (can use pickled) • Green • Shallot • Vidalia/Sweet	• Queso Fresco • Feta • Goat • Mozzarella	• Fava/Lima Bean • Edamame • Chickpea - roasted or drained & rinsed • Black Bean • Kidney Bean	• Black Olive • Kalamata Olive • Artichoke Heart • Heart of Palm • Beet • Arugula • Baby Spinach • Kale	• Pepita/Pumpkin Seed • Sunflower Seed • Pine Nut • Almond - slivered • Pistachio

Dressing

Mix separately, then toss with quinoa before adding other ingredients

Oil *4T; mix neutral + flavored*	**Acid** *4T; can mix vinegar + citrus*	**Fresh Herbs** *2-3 types, plentiful; chopped*	**Salt & Pepper** *both, to taste*	**Chilis** *2 recommended; finely diced*	**Seasonings** *include selectively*
• Avocado • Vegetable • Grapeseed • Olive • Sesame • Chili	• Red Wine Vinegar • Apple Cider Vinegar • Rice Vinegar • Lime Juice • Lemon Juice	• Cilantro • Mint • Oregano • Parsley • Tarragon, Basil • Shiso/Perilla	• Sea Salt • Kosher Salt • Himalayan Salt • Mixed Peppercorn • Black Pepper • White Pepper	• Jalapeño • Serrano • Banana Pepper • Anaheim • Rocotillo	• Red Pepper Flakes • Minced Garlic • Cumin • Yuzu paste

Suggested quantities are per 0.75c dry or 2.25c cooked quinoa. Serves 4-8, as an appetizer or side.

Ingredients flow left to right from essential to optional, and top to bottom from easiest to pair to those needing more consideration.

Tips on how to apply

Getting Started

Stock some quinoa (which has a long shelf life) and be sure to have some type of fresh herbs, veggies, and ideally, queso fresco or feta on hand; frozen corn and edamame are also helpful to keep stocked, so you can whip together a quinoa salad on a moment's notice.

Keeping it Healthy

This is one of the healthiest things you can eat: high in satiating protein and nutrients, while low in fat – just don't go heavy on the oil/cheese.

Pairings & Balance

While most of these ingredients work well with each other, ingredients lower on each list more require consideration on how to pair.

Other Tips

- Shelf Life: Great if made hours or a day in advance and lasts ~2 days refrigerated (keeping the dressing separate helps).
- Other Variations: While less traditional, for a sweeter variation, add fresh/dried fruits, honey or maple syrup.
    - Alternatively, consider adding Meal Prep Chicken or other meat.

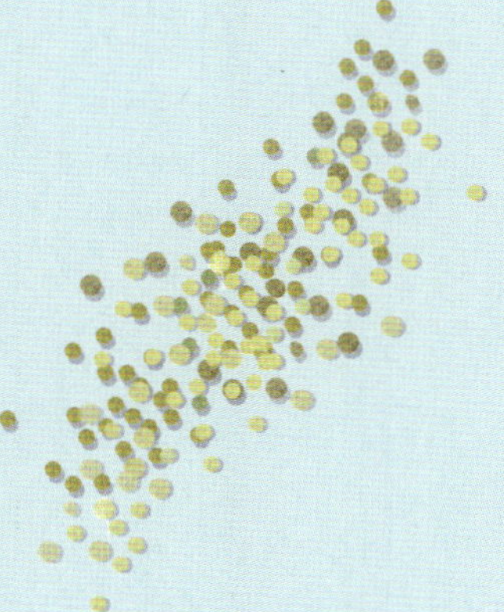

Example pairings

New Classic

Rainbow Quinoa, Cherry Tomato, Bell Pepper, Corn, Avocado, Shallot, Queso Fresco, Edamame, Black Olive

Dressing: Olive Oil, Avocado Oil, White Wine Vinegar, Lime Juice, Cilantro, Mint, Serrano Chili, Banana Pepper

Traditional

Quinoa, Tomato, Corn, Onion, Queso Fresco, Lima Bean, Black Olive

Dressing: Neutral Oil, Vinegar, Parsley, Huacatay, Oregano, Rocoto Chili, Yellow Chili

Japanese

Quinoa, Cherry Tomato, Shishito Pepper, Corn, Avocado, Green Onion, Queso Fresco, Edamame

Dressing: Sesame Oil, Neutral Oil, Rice Vinegar, Shiso, Shichimi Togarashi, Yuzu Paste

Protein

Quinoa, Cherry Tomato, Corn, Avocado, Onion, Queso Fresco, Edamame, Roasted Chickpea, Pepita, Sautéed Chicken

Dressing: Olive Oil, Vinegar, Lime Juice, Cilantro, Mint, Jalapeño

Basic

Quinoa, Tomato, Corn, Onion, Queso Fresco

Dressing: Neutral Oil, Vinegar, Oregano, Red Pepper Flakes; optional: Cilantro

Mediterranean

Quinoa, Tomato, Cucumber, Corn, Avocado, Red Onion, Feta, Baby Spinach, Kalamata Olive

Dressing: Olive Oil, White Wine Vinegar, Lemon Juice, Oregano, Basil

Californian

Rainbow Quinoa, Cherry Tomato, Cucumber, Corn, Avocado, Shallot, Edamame, Black Olive, Arugula

Dressing: Olive Oil, Avocado Oil, Champagne Vinegar, Lime Juice, Cilantro, Mint, Anaheim Chili

Pasta Salad Framework with Soba Variation

Toss pasta into a bold, satisfying salad – or take a soba-inspired path with subtlety and depth.

This framework echoes the Ultimate Salad structure, adapted for a noodle base with rebalanced proportions and priorities. Start with cooked pasta or soba, then layer across categories – both pair well with protein for a more complete meal.

Salad Base

Boil and chill Noodles; combine desired ingredients in bowl

Pasta *1 lb dry; boiled & chilled*	**Fresh Veggies** *1-3 types; chopped*	**Onions** *~1/2; thinly sliced*	**Pickles** *1-3 types; sliced*	**Cheeses** *grated/crumbled*	**Proteins** *recommended; chopped*	**Nuts** *optional; toasted, crushed*
• Fusilli • Farfalle • Orzo • Penne • Rigatoni • Macaroni	• Tomato • Cucumber • Arugula or Spinach • Bell Pepper • Garlic-sautéed: ~ Cremini ~ Broccolini ~ Zucchini • Pea – blanched	• Red (can use pickled) • Green • Vidalia/Sweet • Shallot • Leek *Consider sautéing with olive oil & garlic*	• Sun-dried Tomato • Artichoke • Olive • Pepperoncini • Garlic • Calabrian Chili • Caper • Carrot • Green Bean	• Mozzarella • Parmesan • Pecorino • Burrata • Asiago • Fontina • Feta	• Pepperoni/Salami • Prosciutto • Garbanzo, Cannellini, or Edamame • Chicken – grilled/ roasted/sautéed • Shrimp • Smoked Salmon • Boiled Egg • Tofu	• Pistachio • Almond • Pine Nut • Cashew • Walnut • Macadamia

Dressing

Mix together; pour over salad just before serving

Acid *3T; can mix vinegar + citrus*	**Oil** *equal to or half of Acid*	**Salt** *to taste*	**Pepper** *to taste*	**Herbs** *ideally fresh; chopped*	**Seasonings** *include selectively*
• Red Wine, Sherry Vinegar, White Wine, or Champagne Vinegar • Balsamic Vinegar • Lemon Juice • Orange or Lime Juice	• Olive	• Sea Salt • Kosher Salt • Himalayan Salt	• Mixed Peppercorn • Black Pepper • White Pepper	• Basil • Oregano • Parsley • Tarragon • Thyme • Mint • Cilantro	• Red Pepper Flakes • Minced Garlic • Pesto • Ginger

Suggested quantities are per 1 lb pasta. Serves 4-8, depending on other courses available.

Ingredients flow left to right from essential to optional, and top to bottom from most recommended to those requiring more pairing consideration for Pasta Salad.

Tips on how to apply

Getting Started

You may already have all the ingredients you need - while fusilli and farfalle pastas are most typical, any pasta works. Having a variety of pickles and Italian cured meats will instantly boost your Pasta Salad repertoire.

Keeping it Healthy

Pasta salad can be more balanced than a typical salad, with added protein from meats, cheese, or legumes - it's also higher in carbs and fat, so consider how it fits into your overall meal.

- Pasta: Opt for protein-enriched, whole-grain, or legume-based for extra protein/fiber.
- Protein: Choose lean options like grilled chicken, shrimp, or beans for satiety without excess fat.
- Dressing & Cheese: Go light on heavy dressings, favoring vinaigrettes or yogurt-based sauces.
- Veggies: Load up for volume and nutrients while keeping calories in check.

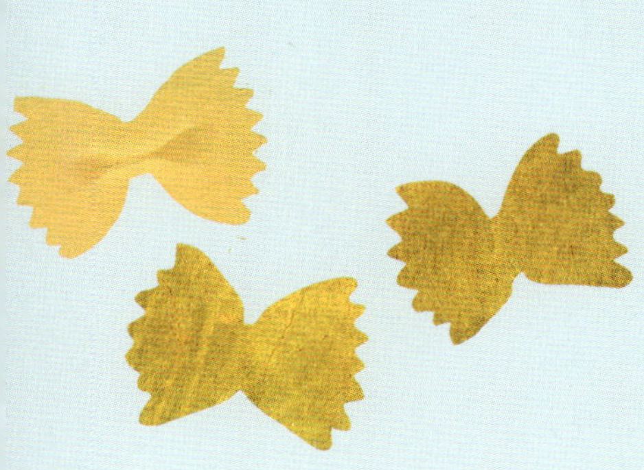

Pairings & Balance

While most of these ingredients work well with each other, ingredients lower on each list more require consideration on how to pair.

Other Tips

- Quantities: Feel free to experiment based on how much you like an ingredient - just remember for strong-flavored ingredients (pickles, nuts), a little goes a long way.
- Chopping: While you can chop to whatever size you see fit, aim to slice/chop ingredients so a knife isn't needed while eating.
- Shelf Life: Great if made hours or a day in advance and lasts ~4 days refrigerated (keeping the dressing separate helps).
- Dressing: Adding some of the brine or oil from the pickles to the dressing is an efficient way to add flavor dimensions and conserve ingredients.

Soba Salad Variation: Follow the same process, substituting chilled soba noodles for pasta and selecting Japanese-inspired ingredients. Try add-ins like Green Onion, Rice Vinegar Pickled Cucumber, Soy Sauce Pickled Shitake, Edamame, Shrimp, and Tofu. For the Dressing, consider Rice Vinegar, Toasted Sesame Oil, Soy Sauce, Togarashi, Shiso, Miso, Bonito, Sesame Seed, and Nori.

Example pairings

Chicken Pesto

Fusilli, Onion, Cherry Tomato, Broccolini, Artichoke Heart, Parmesan, Chopped Sautéed Chicken, Pine Nut

Dressing: White Wine Vinegar, Lemon Juice, Olive Oil, Salt, Pepper, Basil, Minced Garlic, (can supplement with Pesto Sauce, although all ingredients are here)

Classic

Fusilli, Red Onion, Cherry Tomato, Arugula, Pepperoncini, Olive, Mozzarella, Parmesan, Salami

Dressing: White Wine Vinegar, Lemon Juice, Olive Oil, Salt, Pepper, Basil

Orzo Cannellini

Orzo, Vidalia Onion, Garlic-Sautéed Mushroom, Sun-dried Tomato, Cannellini Bean, Pecorino Romano

Dressing: Red Wine Vinegar, Lemon Juice, Olive Oil, Salt, Pepper, Tarragon, Saffron

Smoked Salmon

Penne, Shallot, Cherry Tomato, Arugula, Pea, Fresh Mozzarella, Parmesan, Smoked Salmon

Dressing: White Wine Vinegar, Lemon Zest + Juice, Olive Oil, Salt, Pepper, Parsley, Minced Garlic

Strawberry Balsamic Burrata & Prosciutto 

Farfalle, Red Onion, Tomato, Strawberry, Arugula, Burrata, Prosciutto

Dressing: Balsamic Vinegar, Olive Oil, Salt, Pepper, Basil

Simple Soba Salad 

Soba, Green Onion, Arugula, Boiled Egg; optional: Shiitake (Pickled in Soy Sauce)

Dressing: Rice Vinegar, Sesame Oil, Soy Sauce, Sesame Seed, Nori

Soba Shrimp & Edamame 

Soba, Green Onion, Arugula, Cucumber, Garlic-Ginger Sautéed Shrimp, Edamame

Dressing: Rice Vinegar, Sesame Oil, Soy Sauce, Shichimi Togarashi, Sesame Seed, Nori

Lettuce Wrap Framework

Pack vibrant flavor into every crisp bite with these freestyle-friendly, hand-held salads.

Lettuce wraps thrive on contrast – crisp greens, savory protein, bright herbs, and crunchy toppings. Build across categories to balance texture and flavor, then tie it together with a bold, custom sauce.

Wrap Base

Prepare your fillings, then either wrap in lettuce or arrange everything to assemble as you eat

Base Wrap *3+ large lettuce leaves*	**Proteins** *~0.5 lb total; sautéed*	**Fresh Veggies** *1-3 types; julienne or matchstick*	**Onions** *thinly sliced*	**Pickles** *optional; julienned*	**Herbs** *optional; lightly chopped*	**Nuts & Seeds** *optional; toasted, crushed*
• Romaine • Butter Lettuce • Little Gem • Iceberg • Napa Cabbage • Perilla/Shiso (also serves as Herb)	• Chicken/Turkey - ground • Shrimp • Tofu - marinated • Salmon • Pork - ground • Beef - thinly sliced or ground	• Cucumber • Carrot • Daikon • Snow Pea • Bell Pepper • Jicama • Tomato • Avocado	• Green • Red • Brown - sautéed • Shallot • Crispy Shallot • Pickled Red Onion	• Carrot • Daikon • Kimchi • Quick Pickled Cucumber • Beet • Shiitake • Asian Pear	• Cilantro • Mint • Thai Basil • Green Onion Greens • Perilla/Shiso • Dill	• Peanut • Cashew • Sesame Seed • Sunflower Seed • Almond • Walnut • Pistachio

Build a Sauce

Soy Sauce-Based

Base

- Soy Sauce
- Rice Vinegar

Flavor Boosts

- Garlic, Ginger - minced
- Sesame Oil
- Honey
- Sriracha

Hoisin-Based

Base

- Hoisin Sauce
- Rice Vinegar or Lime Juice

Flavor Boosts

- Garlic - minced
- Sesame Oil
- Sriracha/Sambal

Yogurt-Based

Base

- Plain Greek Yogurt
- Lime Juice or Vinegar

Flavor Boosts

- Garlic - minced
- Mint or Cilantro
- Cucumber - grated

Peanut Sauce

Base

- Peanut Butter + water
- Lime Juice or Vinegar
- Soy Sauce

Flavor Boosts

- Garlic, Ginger - minced
- Honey or Sugar
- Chili Paste

Miso-Based

Base

- Miso Paste + water
- Rice Vinegar

Flavor Boosts

- Ginger - grated
- Honey or Sugar
- Sesame Oil

Fish Sauce (Nước Chấm)

Base

- Fish Sauce + water
- Lime Juice +/– Rice Vinegar

Flavor Boosts

- Sugar
- Garlic - minced
- Chili Paste
- Carrot - shredded

Aim for Vinegar/Citrus juice to be ~1/3 of Base volume; season to taste with salt, and optional Flavor Boosts, adjusting 1-3t at a time

Suggested quantities are per person.

Ingredients flow left to right from essential to optional, and top to bottom from easiest to pair to those needing more consideration.

Tips on how to apply

Getting Started

As long as you have sturdy leafy greens and key sauce ingredients, you can make wraps with just about whatever you have on hand.

- Stocking: Long shelf life items like pickled veggies and nuts add brightness and crunch.
- Sauces: Keep staples like soy sauce, peanut butter, lime, garlic, ginger, and chili on hand to build quick, punchy sauces.

Keeping it Healthy

- This is a naturally healthy dish – just be mindful of sugar/oil in sauces, which is easy to control when making your own.

Pairings & Balance

Wraps are all about contrast – balancing tender proteins with crisp veggies, soft pickles and crunchy nuts. Pair with bold sauces to wow with flavor.

- Herbs: Add brightness and energy – making wraps feel incredibly fresh.
- Acid: Use lime juice to punch up freshness, or rice vinegar to round out savory notes.

Other Tips

- Sauce Building: Start with a base – each works well alone – then add flavor boosts as desired.
    - Dilution: For Peanut Sauce, add water for a pourable consistency; for Miso and Fish Sauce-bases, it helps soften intensity.
- Assembly: Drizzle sauce over the filling or serve on the side for dipping.
- Portioning: Keep filling to ~1/3 of leaf for easier wrapping and eating.
- Serving: Serve open-faced or gently folded – no need to fully enclose.

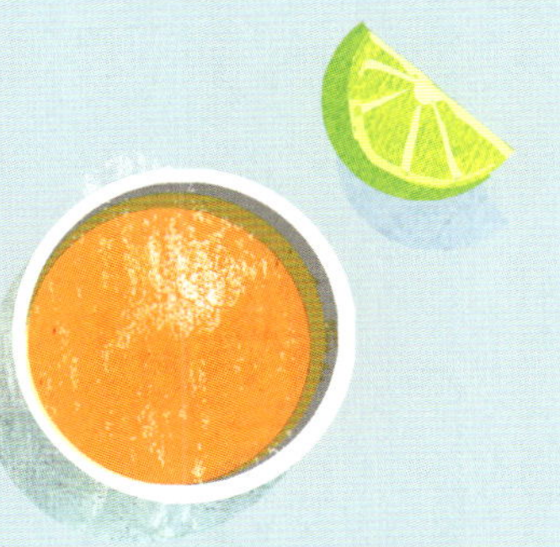

Example pairings

Thai Chicken

Butter Lettuce, Ground Chicken (seasoned with Soy Sauce and Ginger), Cilantro, Green Onion, Snap Pea, Pickled Carrot, Crushed Peanut

Sauce: Peanut-Lime-Garlic-Chil

Shrimp & Herb

Butter Lettuce, Shrimp, Cucumber, Pickled Carrot, Green Onion, Thai Basil, Crispy Shallot

Sauce: Soy-Sauce-Vinegar-Garlic

Ginger Garlic Pork

Napa Cabbage, Ground Pork (sautéed with Garlic and Ginger), Daikon, Bell Pepper, Cilantro, Mint, Cashew

Sauce: Hoisin-Vinegar-Garlic-Sesame Oil

Salmon & Herb

Little Gem, Salmon, Cucumber, Pickled Red Onion, Dill or Mint; optional: Perilla

Sauce: Yogurt-Lime-Garlic-Mint

Korean Beef

Romaine, Beef (sautéed with Soy Sauce, Garlic, and Sesame Oil), Kimchi, Green Onion, Perilla, Sesame Seed

Sauce: Miso-Vinegar-Ginger-Honey

Miso Tofu

Butter Lettuce, Tofu (seared with Soy Sauce and Miso), Carrot, Pickled Daikon, Thai Basil, Peanut

Sauce: Soy Sauce-Vinegar-Chili-Sesame Oil

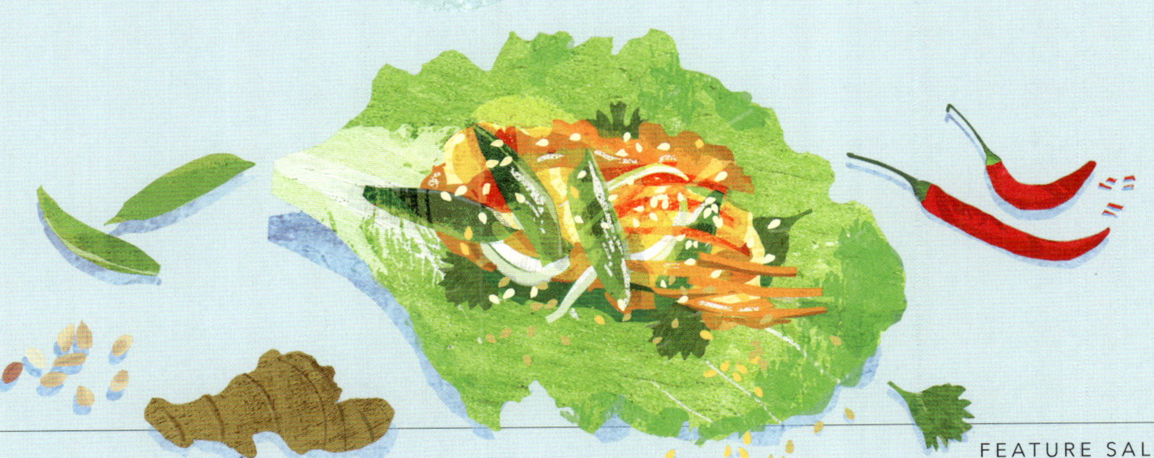

Bowls & Boards

Grain Bowl

Hawaiian Protein Bowl

Charcuterie Board

Antipasto Platter

Picnic Basket

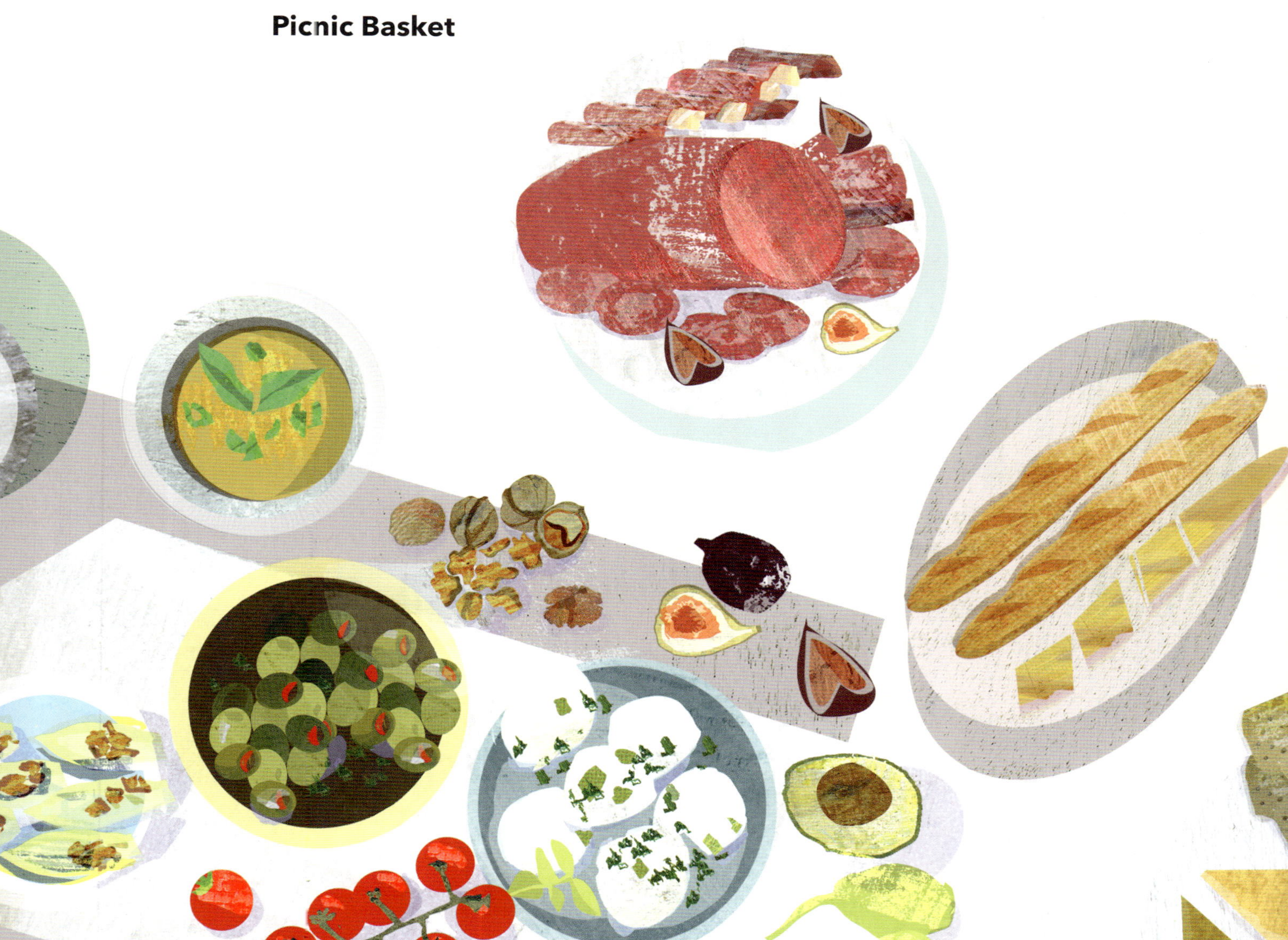

This chapter is all about demystification and inspiration. If you've never assembled a Charcuterie Board or Antipasto Platter before, these frameworks show just how simple it can be – and if you have, they offer quick reference points to level up your approach with new flair and more thoughtful pairings.

It's also one of the most social chapters in this book – these dishes naturally invite sharing, interaction, and creativity. Whether you're plating a board for two or prepping ingredients for an impromptu grain bowl bar, they're flexible enough to suit any setting.

The pinnacle of this spirit is the Picnic Basket: a timeless tradition worth reviving. It's a gentle reminder that food doesn't have to be fussy to be meaningful – and that sometimes, the best meals are shared on a blanket under the trees.

Grain Bowl Framework

Build satisfying, layered bowls where hearty grains and bold proteins take center stage.

Think of grain bowls as an evolution of salads – with grains as the base and greater emphasis on protein. The pairing intuition you built in earlier frameworks still applies: build across categories to create contrast and depth.

Base

Combine desired ingredients in bowl

Grains *~0.5c cooked; chilled*	**Proteins** *~0.5 lb; chopped*	**Leafy Greens & Onions** *1 of each category*	**Fresh Veggies** *1-3 types; chopped*	**Roasted Veggies** *0-2 types; chopped*	**Pickles** *optional; sliced*	**Nuts & Seeds** *optional; toasted, crushed*
• Farro • Barley • Quinoa • Brown Rice • Bulgur	• Chicken – grilled • Salmon – seared/ grilled • Tuna – seared/ canned • Egg – boiled • Edamame • Chickpea – roasted or drained & rinsed • Tofu – roasted	• Arugula • Baby Spinach • Kale • Cabbage – shredded --- • Green Onion • Red Onion • Shallot	• Tomato • Bell Pepper • Avocado • Cucumber • Carrot – shredded • Corn – steamed • Pea, Snow Pea – blanched	• Sweet Potato • Brussels Sprout • Bell Pepper • Cauliflower • Eggplant • Mushroom • Fennel • Zucchini	• Red Onion • Radish • Kimchi • Artichoke Heart • Olive • Heart of Palm • Beet	• Almond • Pistachio • Cashew • Sunflower Seed • Pepita/Pumpkin Seed • Sesame Seed • Pine Nut

Dressing

Mix together; pour over salad just before serving

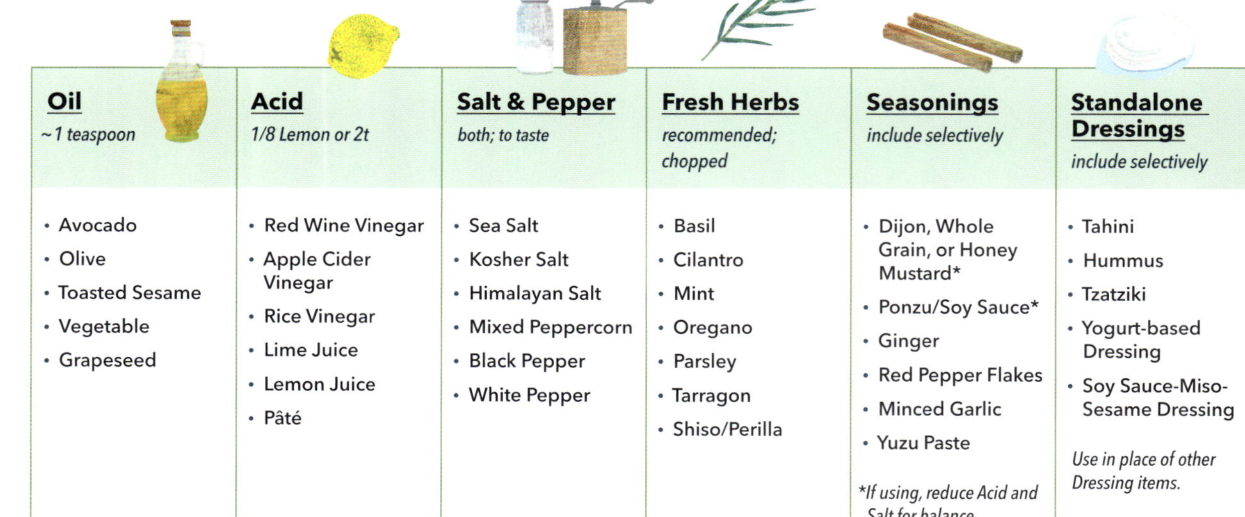

Oil *~1 teaspoon*	**Acid** *1/8 Lemon or 2t*	**Salt & Pepper** *both; to taste*	**Fresh Herbs** *recommended; chopped*	**Seasonings** *include selectively*	**Standalone Dressings** *include selectively*
• Avocado • Olive • Toasted Sesame • Vegetable • Grapeseed	• Red Wine Vinegar • Apple Cider Vinegar • Rice Vinegar • Lime Juice • Lemon Juice • Pâté	• Sea Salt • Kosher Salt • Himalayan Salt • Mixed Peppercorn • Black Pepper • White Pepper	• Basil • Cilantro • Mint • Oregano • Parsley • Tarragon • Shiso/Perilla	• Dijon, Whole Grain, or Honey Mustard* • Ponzu/Soy Sauce* • Ginger • Red Pepper Flakes • Minced Garlic • Yuzu Paste **If using, reduce Acid and Salt for balance.*	• Tahini • Hummus • Tzatziki • Yogurt-based Dressing • Soy Sauce-Miso-Sesame Dressing *Use in place of other Dressing items.*

Suggested quantities are per person.

Ingredients flow left to right from essential to optional, and top to bottom from most recommended to those needing more pairing consideration.

Tips on how to apply

Getting Started

Ensure you have grains, protein and some veggies - the rest is optional or staples - level up with some roasted veggies.

Keeping it Healthy

- Focus on Whole Grains: Use quinoa, brown rice, or farro for added fiber and nutrients.
- Go Heavy on Veggies: Aim to fill half your bowl with fresh or roasted vegetables.
- Lean Proteins: Choose options like grilled chicken, tofu, or legumes to keep it light.
- Limit Heavy Dressings: Use olive oil, lemon juice, or yogurt-based dressings instead of creamy, calorie-dense sauces.

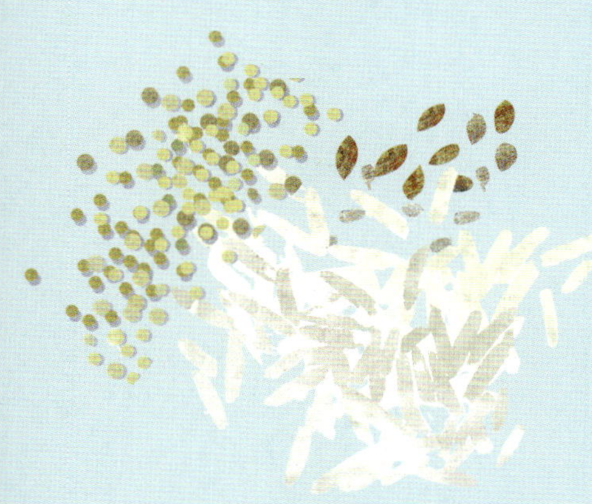

Pairings & Balance

Aim for a mix of savory, sweet, tangy, and spicy in each bowl.

- Layer Textures: Combine creamy (avocado), crunchy (nuts/seeds), and chewy (grains).
- Sweet & Savory: Pair roasted sweet potatoes or dried cranberries with tangy feta or pickled onions.
- Creamy & Crunchy: Balance creamy elements like avocado or tahini with crunchy nuts, seeds, or crispy chickpeas.
- Tangy & Umami: Combine a tangy vinaigrette with umami-rich toppings like miso, soy sauce, or roasted mushrooms.
- Spicy & Mild: Add a kick with chili flakes or sriracha, and balance with cooling cucumbers or yogurt dressing.

Other Tips

- Batch Cook Grains: Cook a big batch of grains and refrigerate for up to 5 days to save time during the week.
- Encore: Grain bowls are perfect for using up leftover veggies, proteins, or sauces from other meals.

Example pairings

Mediterranean Chicken Quinoa

Quinoa, Grilled Chicken, Arugula, Red Onion, Cucumber, Cherry Tomatoes, Roasted Eggplant, Kalamata Olive, Pine Nut

Dressing: Lemon-Tahini-Garlic

Middle Eastern

Couscous, Falafel, Leafy Green Mix, Pickled Red Onion, Cucumber, Cherry Tomato, Roasted Zucchini, Almond

Dressing: Yogurt-Cucumber (with Garlic, Lemon Juice)

Autumn Salmon

Wild Rice, Grilled Salmon, Red Onion, Corn, Cucumber, Pickled Beet, Roasted Brussels Sprout, Pumpkin Seed

Dressing: Balsamic Vinaigrette*

Fall Harvest

Farro, Roasted Turkey, Baby Kale, Sautéed Shallot, Apple, Roasted Acorn Squash, Dried Cranberry, Pecan

Dressing: Maple-Dijon Vinaigrette

Thai Shrimp

Jasmine Rice, Shrimp, Shredded Cabbage, Green Onion, Carrot, Bell Pepper, Pickled Cucumber (Rice Vinegar, Sugar, Salt), Peanut, Cilantro

Dressing: Spicy Peanut Sauce (prepared or Peanut Butter, Lime Juice, Rice Vinegar, Soy Sauce, Water, Garlic, Sugar, Ginger, Sriracha)

Vegan Power Protein 

Quinoa, Roasted Chickpea, Spinach, Red Onion, Cherry Tomato, Cucumber, Roasted Sweet Potato, Cauliflower, Pickled Radish, Chia Seed

Dressing: Lemon-Tahini-Garlic

***Vinaigrette** 1-3 parts olive oil to 1 part vinegar/ lemon juice + salt & pepper

Hawaiian Protein Bowl Framework

Bring tropical energy to your bowl with tangy marinades, juicy proteins, and bright, balanced toppings.

This framework flips the typical salad/bowl structure, starting with a sauce: whisk together oil, acid, sweet, herbs, and prepared sauces to marinate the protein while prepping the other ingredients. Grill or sauté protein (or use pre-cooked meal prep) before assembling your bowl with rice, veggies, and more.

Marinade/Sauce

Mix ingredients; use half to marinate the protein and drizzle the rest over the bowl before serving.

Prepared Sauces *1-3T combined*	**Acid** *~1T*	**Oil** *~2 t*	**Sweet** *0-1T*	**Herbs** *1T +garnish*	**Seasonings** *0.5-1T*
• Soy Sauce/Ponzu • Teriyaki • Sesame Sauce • Mayo +/- Sriracha • Hoisin • Miso Paste • Yuzu Paste	• Rice Vinegar • Lime Juice • Lemon Juice • Yuzu Juice	• Sesame • Toasted Sesame • Avocado • Other Neutral Oil • Olive • Chili	• Brown Sugar • Honey • Raw Sugar • Sugar • Mirin • Pineapple Juice • Maple Syrup	• Cilantro • Mint • Thai Basil • Shiso/Perilla • Nori • Chives	• Furikake • Togarashi • Ginger - grated or pickled • Minced Garlic • Five-Spice • Red Pepper Flakes • Smoked Paprika

Base

Prepare Rice and Protein; combine desired ingredients in bowl

Rice *~0.5c cooked; chilled*	**Proteins** *~0.5 lb total; sliced*	**Leafy Greens & Onions** *1 of each category*	**Fresh Veggies** *1-3 types; chopped*	**Pickles** *1-2 types; sliced*	**Fruits** *optional; sliced*	**Nuts & Seeds** *optional; toasted, crushed*
• White Rice (Calrose or Sushi Rice) • Brown • Red • Black	• Chicken • Shrimp • Pork Tenderloin or Char Siu-style • Spam • Salmon • Tofu • Edamame - steamed	• Baby Spinach • Arugula • Spring Mix • Romaine --- • Green Onion • Sweet Onion • Shallot	• Cucumber • Carrot - shredded • Bell Pepper • Snap Pea • Tomato • Water Chestnut • Watermelon Radish • Jicama	• Quick Pickled Cucumber • Red Onion • Kimchi • Daikon • Carrot • Jalapeño • Mango	• Mango • Pineapple • Papaya • Avocado • Orange • Strawberry • Kiwi • Starfruit	• Macadamia • Cashew • Peanut • Sesame Seed • Almond • Pistachio

Suggested quantities are per person.

Ingredients flow left to right from essential to optional, and top to bottom from most recommended to those needing more pairing consideration.

Tips on how to apply

Getting Started

Keep rice, rice vinegar, and soy sauce on hand, along with sesame oil, nori, and frozen edamame, and you'll always be close to a great bowl. Then just pick up your preferred protein and fresh veggies.

Keeping it Healthy

These bowls are naturally health-forward - dial it even further with:

- Veggies: Aim to fill at least half the bowl with fresh and pickled vegetables.
- Protein: Include plant-based protein such as edamame.
- Mayo: Go easy on mayo-based sauces.
- Rice: Brown or red rice offers a more sustained energy release than white.

Pairings & Balance:

Ingredients here are made to mix and match - aim for visual contrast and texture variety. Combine crisp and tender, fresh and pickled, soft and crunchy (e.g., nuts, fried shallots, water chestnuts).

- Oil: Use a 50/50 mix of sesame and a neutral oil to keep sesame from overpowering.

Sauce Adjustments

- Ponzu: Basically 45% soy sauce, 45% vinegar/citrus juice, 10% mirin, so adjust those proportionally.
- Teriyaki: Primarily soy sauce and sugar, so reduce those if using it.
- Mirin: If skipping, increase rice vinegar and sugar slightly to balance.

Other Tips

- Simplicity: There are countless ingredient options - start with your favorites.
- Social Spread: For groups, consider preparing ingredients each in their own bowl, so guests can assemble their own - this saves time and creates a fun, social experience.
- Sriracha Mayo: Simply mix 50/50 sriracha and (Japanese) mayo.

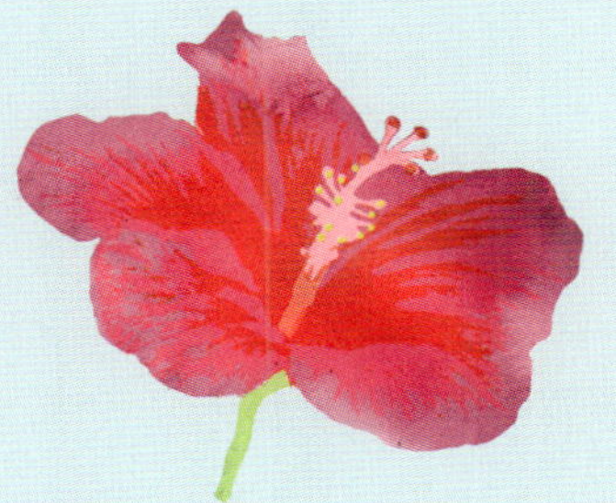

Example pairings

Teriyaki Chicken

Marinate: Chicken, Teriyaki Sauce, Rice Vinegar, Sesame Oil, Ginger; then grill or pan-fry

Accompany: Avocado, Cucumber Salad, Edamame, Shredded Carrot

Garnish: Green Onion, Sesame Seeds

Garlic Ginger Shrimp

Marinate: Shrimp, Soy Sauce, Rice Vinegar, Olive Oil, Honey, Garlic, Ginger, Mirin; then sauté

Accompany: Avocado, Cherry Tomato

Garnish: Green Onion, Nori, Sesame Seeds

Citrus Miso Salmon

Marinate: Salmon, White Miso, Lime Juice, Soy Sauce, Sesame Oil, Garlic; then grill or sauté

Accompany: Cucumber, (pickled) Mango, Avocado, Red Onion

Garnish: Green Onion, Toasted Sesame Seed

Charred Spam & Pineapple

Marinate: Spam, charred briefly in a pan/grill

Accompany: Grilled Pineapple, Shredded Lettuce, Pickled Cucumber, Tomato

Garnish: Green Onion, Furikake, Macadamia

Spicy Pork & Kimchi

Marinate: Pork Tenderloin, Gochujang, Rice Vinegar, Garlic, Ginger; then sauté

Accompany: Cucumber, Kimchi, Pickled Daikon, Avocado

Garnish: Green Onion, Toasted Sesame Seec

Citrus Soy Tofu

Marinate: Tofu, Soy Sauce, Lime Juice, Sesame Oil, Garlic, Chili Flakes; then sauté

Accompany: Shredded Cabbage, Mandarin Orange Slices, Pickled Red Onion, Edamame

Garnish: Mint, Macadamia

Charcuterie Board Framework

Consider your board a blank canvas: visualize your design, place key ingredients first, then artfully fill spaces using your palette of flavors.

Mix flavors, textures, and colors across categories to design balanced boards, selecting a few items from each to create contrast and variety. This framework is highly adaptable, letting you mix and match components based on preferences, occasion, or what's on hand.

Ingredients

Cured Meats *2+ types; mix textures*	**Cheeses** *~1 per category*	**Fresh Fruits** *1+ type; bite-sized*	**Dried Fruits** *1+ type; whole*	**Nuts & Seeds** *1+ type; toasted*	**Pickles** *[optional]*	**Veggies** *[optional]*
• Prosciutto • Salami (Soppressata, Calabrese, Genoa) • Jamón Serrano • Spanish Chorizo • Coppa • Duck Prosciutto	• Hard: Gruyère, Manchego, Aged Cheddar, Parmesan • Semi-Soft: Havarti, Fontina, Blue • Soft: Goat, Brie, Camembert • Flavored: Herb-crusted Goat, Smoked Gouda	• Grape • Strawberry • Fig • Pear - sliced • Apple - sliced • Blackberry • Raspberry • Blueberry	• Apricot • Date • Fig • Peach • Cranberry • Raisin • Prune	• Almond - roasted/smoked • Walnut • Pistachio • Cashew • Macadamia • Pecan • Pepita/Pumpkin Seed	• Cornichons • Olive • Onion • Carrot • Artichoke • Sun-dried Tomato • Pimiento • Banana Pepper	• Bell Pepper - spears • Cherry Tomato • Carrot - spears • Cucumber - sliced • Snap Pea • Broccoli • Mushroom (Garlic-Sautéed) • Celery

Accompaniments

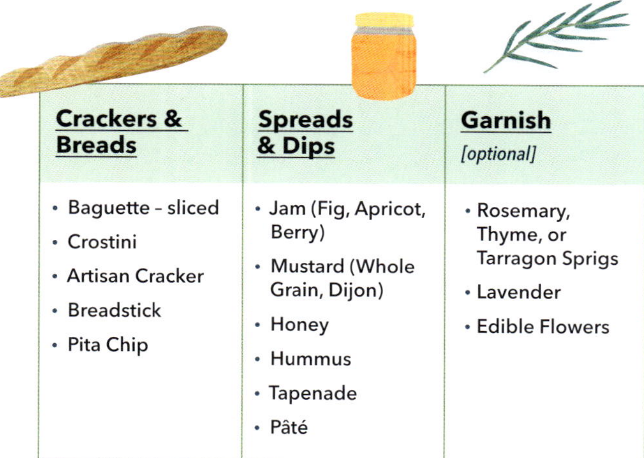

Crackers & Breads	**Spreads & Dips**	**Garnish** *[optional]*
• Baguette - sliced • Crostini • Artisan Cracker • Breadstick • Pita Chip	• Jam (Fig, Apricot, Berry) • Mustard (Whole Grain, Dijon) • Honey • Hummus • Tapenade • Pâté	• Rosemary, Thyme, or Tarragon Sprigs • Lavender • Edible Flowers

Key Equipment

- Cheese Knife
- Spreading Knife
- Toothpicks

Aim for 2-3 oz of meat and 2-3 oz cheese per person, with additional items filling out the rest.

Ingredients flow left to right from essential to optional, and top to bottom from most recommended to those needing more pairing consideration.

Tips on how to apply

Getting Started

If you've stocked up on dried fruits, nuts, pickles, cured meats and hard cheese from earlier frameworks, you could probably whip together a charcuterie board on a whim – pick up some fresh fruits, soft/semi-soft cheese, and perhaps some fresh veggies to level up.

Keeping it Healthy

- Include plenty of fresh fruits and vegetables to lighten the board.
- Whole-Grain: Crackers/bread for added fiber.
- Include Plant-Based Protein: Add roasted chickpeas, hummus, or spiced nuts for variety and a healthier protein boost.

Pairings & Balance

Pair salty cured meats with sweet fruits like figs or honey for contrast and offset creamy cheeses with tangy items like pickled onion or cornichons.

- Texture: Combine crunchy nuts or breadsticks with soft spreads or cheeses to keep each bite interesting.

Other Tips

- Prevent Discoloration: Add a bit of lime or lemon juice to apple and pear slices.
- Pre-Cut and Serve: Pre-slice cheeses and meats for easy serving and an approachable presentation.
- Temperature: Let cheeses come to room temperature for the best flavor and texture; keep meats chilled until serving.
- Board Arrangement: Place larger items (like cheeses and bowls of dips) first, then fill in with smaller items for a balanced layout. Choose a focal point (such as a premium cheese or unique cured meat) and build the board around it.
- Seasonal Themes: Tailor to the season. Add citrus and pomegranate seeds in winter or berries and edible flowers in spring.

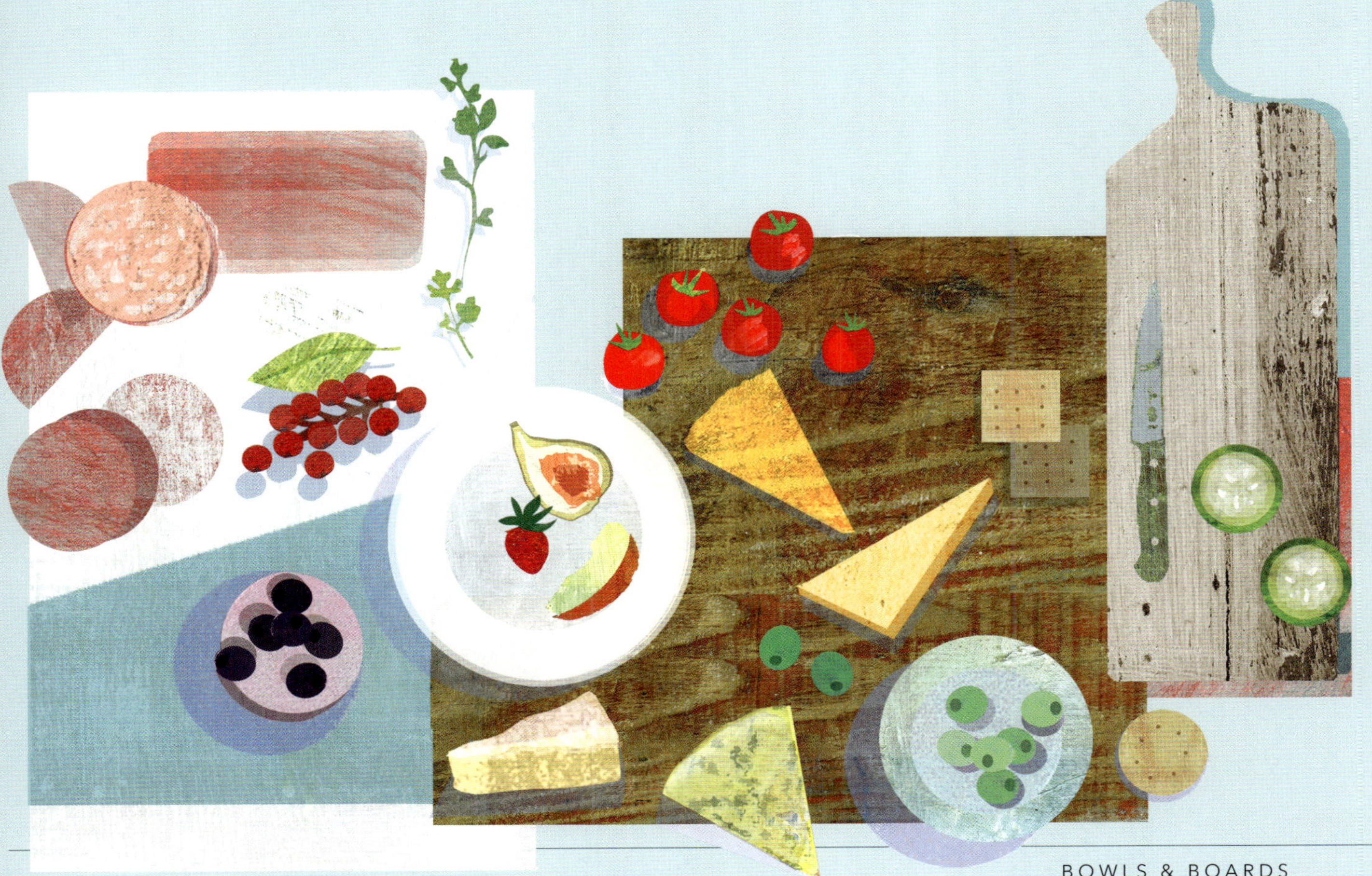

Antipasto Platter Framework

Think of your platter as a landscape: anchor it with key ingredients first, then thoughtfully cluster complementary items around them.

This framework echoes the Charcuterie Board, leaning Italian and Greek with a stronger focus on marinated and fresh vegetables. Mix flavors, textures, and colors across categories, selecting a few items from each to create contrast and balance.

Ingredients

Cured Meats *2+ types; mix textures*	**Cheeses** *2+ types; mix textures*	**Marinated Veggies** *2+ types*	**Fresh Veggies** *2+ types; bite-sized/ spears*	**Pickles** *1+ type; bite-sized*	**Nuts** *1+ type; toasted, shelled*	**Fruits** *1+ type; whole*
• Prosciutto • Bresaola • Salami (Soppressata, Calabrese, Genoa, Mortadella) • Jamón Serrano • Chorizo Ibérico • Coppa • Duck Prosciutto	• Hard: Pecorino, Parmigiano-Reggiano, Asiago, Aged Gouda • Semi-Soft: Fontina, Provolone, Smoked Scamorza • Soft: Mozzarella, Burrata, Ricotta	• Sun-dried Tomato • Roasted Red Pepper • Artichoke • Olive • Mushroom (Garlic-sautéed) • Eggplant Caponata • Dolma	• Cherry Tomato • Bell Pepper • Cucumber • Endive • Carrot • Celery • Broccoli	• Giardiniera (Italian Pickled Vegetables) • Pepperoncini • Onion • Carrot • Caper • Beet	• Almond - marinated/ roasted • Pistachio • Walnut • Pine Nut • Cashew • Hazelnut	• Grape • Fig (fresh or dried) • Apricot (dried) • Date • Cranberry (dried) • Cherry (fresh or dried) • Golden Raisin

Accompaniments

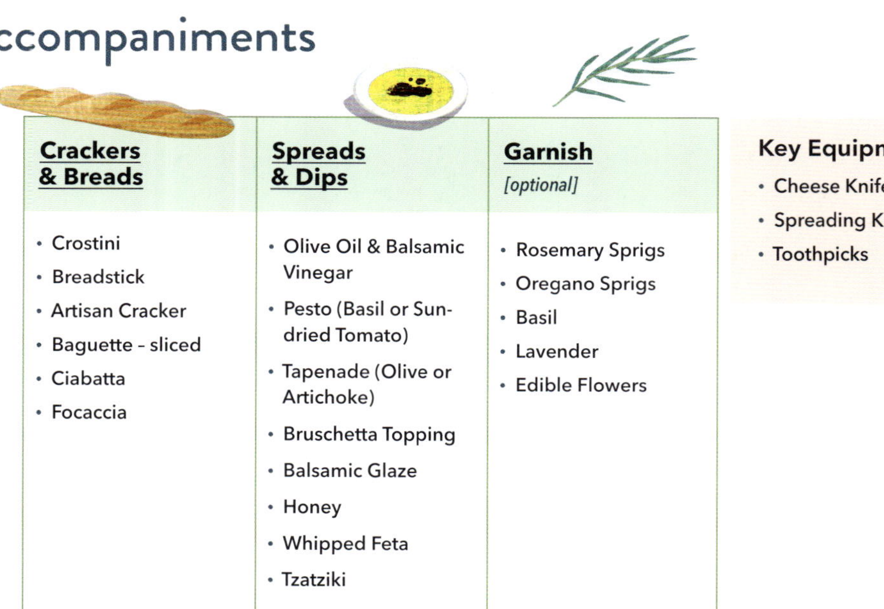

Crackers & Breads	**Spreads & Dips**	**Garnish** *[optional]*
• Crostini • Breadstick • Artisan Cracker • Baguette - sliced • Ciabatta • Focaccia	• Olive Oil & Balsamic Vinegar • Pesto (Basil or Sun-dried Tomato) • Tapenade (Olive or Artichoke) • Bruschetta Topping • Balsamic Glaze • Honey • Whipped Feta • Tzatziki	• Rosemary Sprigs • Oregano Sprigs • Basil • Lavender • Edible Flowers

Key Equipment

- Cheese Knife
- Spreading Knife
- Toothpicks

Aim for 2-3 oz of meat and 2-3 oz cheese per person, with additional items filling out the rest.

Ingredients flow left to right from essential to optional, and top to bottom from most recommended to those needing more pairing consideration.

Tips on how to apply

Getting Started

If you've stocked up on dried fruits, nuts, pickled/marinated veggies, cured meats and hard cheese from earlier frameworks, you could probably whip together an Antipasto platter on a whim – pick up some fresh veggies, fruits, and additional cheese to level up.

Keeping it Healthy

Focus on fresh and marinated veggies to lighten the platter.

- Meat: Check the label for fat content or select meets with less visible white fat.
- Cheese: Check the label for fat content per serving.

Pairings & Balance

Combine fatty meats and cheeses with acidic pickles or marinated veggies to balance the richness.

- Spreads: Offer a sweet (e.g., honey) and a savory (e.g., pesto) spread for versatility.
- Seasonal Themes: Incorporate seasonal produce like fresh figs in the summer or citrus in the winter.

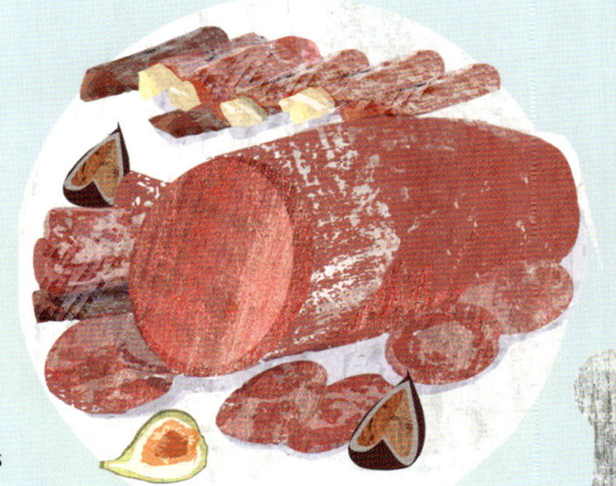

Other Tips

- Pre-Cut and Serve: Pre-slice cheeses and meats for easy serving and an approachable presentation.
- Temperature: Let meats and cheeses sit out for 15-30 min before serving for optimal flavor.
- Presentation: Arrange items in clusters or flowing lines for visual appeal.

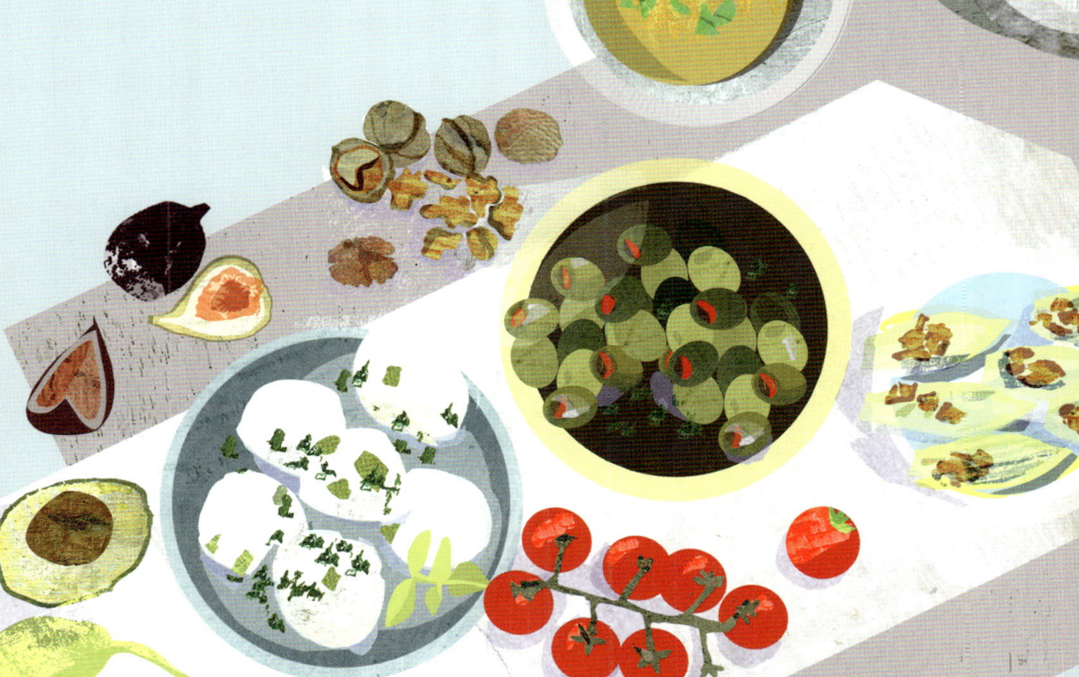

Picnic Basket Framework

Revive a timeless tradition by bringing impromptu assemblages into nature for memorable experiences with those you cherish.

Select a few items across categories to build a portable spread with contrast, comfort, and character. Think balance - something creamy, something crunchy, something fresh - all easy to transport and enjoy outdoors.

Ingredients

Bread & Crackers *1-2 types*	**Cheeses** *mix textures*	**Proteins** *1-2 types; sliceable/ bite-size*	**Fruits** *1-2 types; mix textures*	**Veggies** *1-2 types; fresh or pickled*	**Nuts** *[optional]*	**Spreads & Dips** *[optional]*
• Baguette • Crostini • Multigrain Cracker • Water Cracker • Flatbread/Pita • Breadstick/ Grissini	• Firm: Aged Cheddar, Manchego, Gouda • Soft: Goat Cheese, Brie, Ricotta	• Prosciutto • Salami • Spanish Chorizo • Chicken - grilled • Meatball • Boiled Egg • Marinated Tofu • Caviar	• Grape • Strawberry • Blackberry • Apple • Peach • Fig (fresh or dried) • Apricot (dried) • Date	• Cherry Tomato • Snap Pea • Cucumber - spears • Bell Pepper - spears • Carrot - spears • Gherkin • Olive • Sun-dried Tomato	• Almond - marinated/ roasted • Cashew • Pistachio • Sunflower Seed • Candied Nuts	• Jam/Marmalade • Tapenade • Hummus • Eggplant Spread • Yogurt Dip • Honey • Pâté

Accompaniments

Hearty Salads: *optional; store-bought or from scratch*	**Sweets** *[optional]*	**Beverages** *[optional]*
• Grain: Farro/Quinoa, Cucumber, Cherry Tomato, Parsley, Mint, Feta, Red Onion, Olive Oil, Lemon Juice, Seasoning • Lentil: Lentil, Carrot, Fennel, Red Onion or Shallot, Parsley, Olive Oil, Red Wine Vinegar, Seasoning • Roasted Veggie: Roasted Sweet Potato and Carrot, Arugula, Goat Cheese, toasted Nuts, Olive Oil, Lemon Juice, Seasoning • Marinated Mushroom: Mushroom (marinated with Red Onion, Vinegar, Olive Oil, Garlic), Parsley, Seasoning • Chickpea: Roasted Chickpea, Cucumber, Tomato, Red Onion, Parsley, Feta, Olive Oil, Lemon Juice, Seasoning • Pasta Salad: See earlier framework (p20)	• Cookies • Brownies • Chocolate • Chocolate-Dipped Fruit • Honey • Peanut Brittle • Madeleines • Marzipan *Opt for firm items that travel well.*	• Water (sparkling or flavored) • Wine/Sangria • Champagne • Tea (hot or iced) • Coffee • Juice/Lemonade • Fruit Soda

Key Equipment

- Basket or Cooler Bag
- Cups, Plates, Utensils
- Blanket or Tablecloth
- Cutting Board & Knife
- Thermos
- Napkins
- Corkscrew

Aim for 6 oz+ of Cheese and 6 oz+ Protein per person, with additional items filling out the rest.

Ingredients flow left to right from essential to optional, and top to bottom from most recommended to those needing more pairing consideration.

Tips on how to apply

Getting Started

Whether you're using a formal picnic basket, a padded tote, or a cooler bag, once you've got the container, you'll be surprised how much can come straight from your pantry - nuts, dried fruit, cured meats, hard cheeses, even jams or dips. From there, just pick up a few fresh items like fruit and bread to round out the spread.

Keeping it Healthy

Feature fresh veggies and lean into fruit as your main dessert.

- Cheese: Check the label if you're aiming to keep it light - fat content can vary widely.
- Beverages: Consider tea, juice or sparkling sodas with a high percentage of real fruit juice and minimal added sugar - commercial iced tea/lemonade can be high in sugar.

Pairings & Balance

The beauty of a picnic spread is how easily it all mixes and matches - just aim to represent a few different categories (e.g., something salty, something crunchy, something fresh, something creamy) for a well-rounded experience.

Other Tips

- Pre-Cutting: Slice bread, meats, and cheese ahead to have a more relaxed picnic - or leave some to slice in the moment to keep fresh and extend the meal.
- Packing: Use small containers for spreads, dips, and nuts; wrap cheeses in parchment for easy unpacking; bring ice if anything needs to stay chilled.
- Safety: Wrap any sharp knives in a napkin or towel and secure with a rubber band.
- Sourcing: This can be worth a splurge at a specialty grocery or cheese counter - or you can absolutely build a beautiful basket from any well-stocked grocery store.
- Flair: Even a single flower or sprig of herbs (like lavender or rosemary) adds a photogenic touch and elegant charm.
- Encore: Incorporate any surplus picnic ingredients to elevate future salads with gourmet flair.

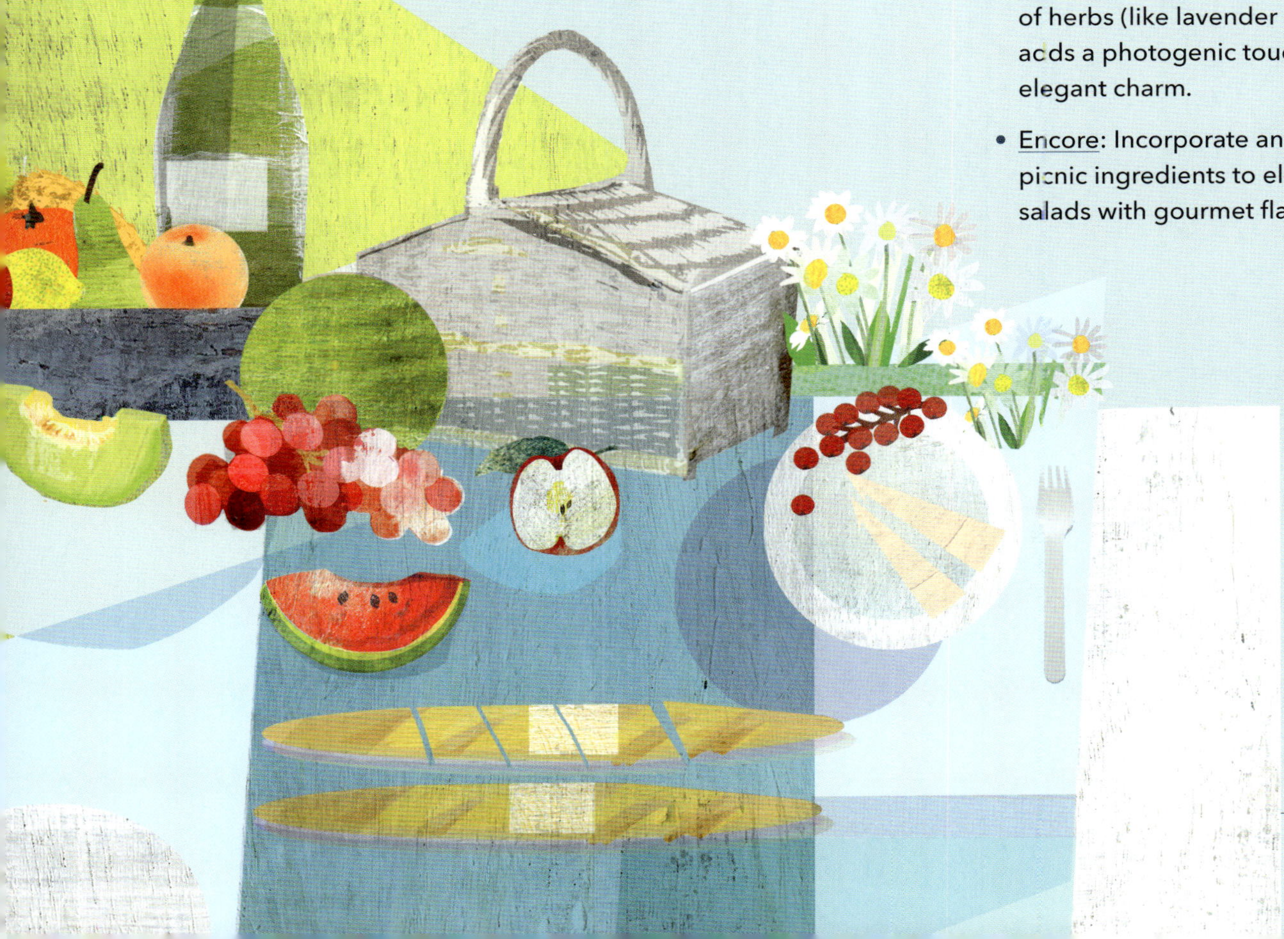

Breakfast & Brunch

Smoothie

Açaí Bowl

Overnight Oats

Scrambled Egg

Omelet

Frittata

Shakshuka

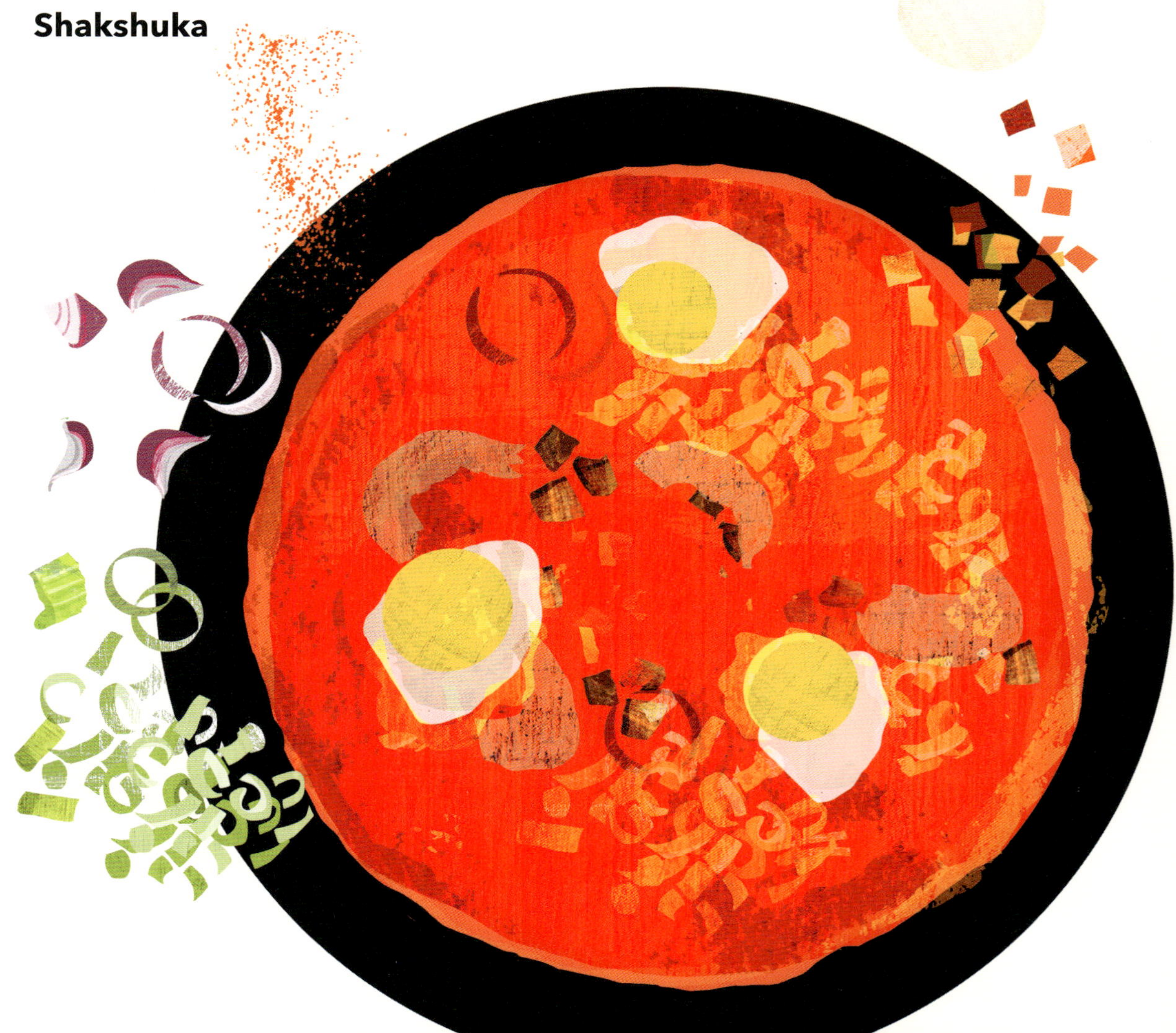

Breakfast and brunch are where improvisation shines. These dishes are quick to make, endlessly adaptable, and forgiving – perfect for testing out new flavors, techniques, and pairings. Whether you're cooking for a crowd or just yourself, this is where confidence in the kitchen is built.

Each framework in this section takes on a unique, infographic look, making it easy to experiment and refine your skills.

Pick a dish and commit to making it a few times with different variations. The first time: it will work. The second time: you'll impress others. By the third: you'll impress yourself – turning a simple concept into a personal masterpiece of culinary innovation.

Smoothie Framework

Think of Smoothies as a blended salad – choose ingredients spanning categories while balancing frozen, liquid, and (optional) solid components.

Think texture first, flavor second. Start with frozen to chill, then pour in enough liquid to get it blending. From there, toss in anything that excites you: fresh fruits, greens, supplements, even spices. If it sounds good together in your head, it should work in the blender.

Solid

Add as desired and adjust Liquid for desired consistency

Fresh Fruit

- Any of below fruits or Kiwi, Grape, Pear, Melon

Yogurt

- Low/Non-fat, Vanilla, Plain or Fruit-flavored

Supplements

- Protein Powder (Vanilla, Chocolate, etc.)
- Green Power Powder, Chia/Flaxseed
- Creatine, Matcha Powder, Pre-workout

Veggies

- Spinach, Kale, Tomato, Carrot, Celery, Cauliflower

Spices*

- Ginger Powder, Cardamom, Mint, Vanilla Extract, Cinnamon, Nutmeg, Turmeric

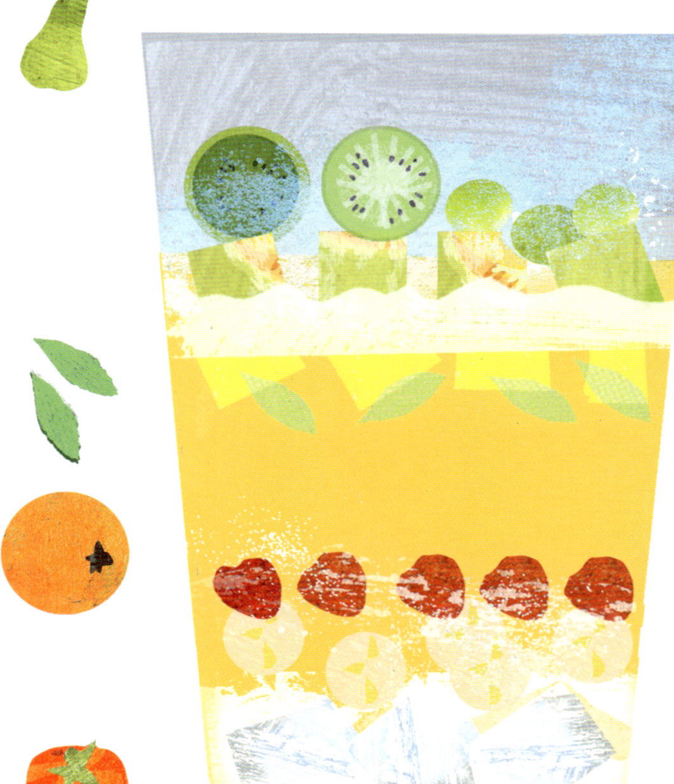

Liquid

Add as needed to purée, roughly matching Frozen volume

Fruit Juice

- Orange, Apple, Pomegranate*, Guava

Dairy

- Almond Milk (Plain, Vanilla), Milk, Oat Milk, Coconut Milk

Water, etc.

- Water, Coconut Water, Iced Tea, Kombucha, Coffee (chilled)

Veggie Juice

- Carrot, Beet, Tomato, V8 or other blend

Frozen

Crush ~1c in blender

Frozen Fruits

- Banana, Strawberry, Mango, Peach, Açaí, Blueberry, Blackberry, Raspberry, Pineapple, Cherry

Frozen Yogurt

- Low/Non-fat, Vanilla, Plain or Fruit-flavored

Ice

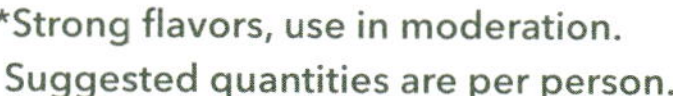

*Strong flavors, use in moderation.
Suggested quantities are per person.

Ingredients flow from easiest to pair to those inviting more creative consideration.

Tips on how to apply

Getting Started

Stock up on vanilla protein powder and frozen fruits like strawberries, peach, mango, and pineapple. Keep bananas, (unsweetened vanilla almond) milk, and orange juice on hand to enable a range of blends.

Keeping it Healthy

Keep your smoothies from becoming sugar bombs by using a moderate amount of fruit, add flavor with protein powder, and use water/ice to reach the right consistency; add a scoop of green power powder to make it even more nutrient-dense, without dramatically altering flavor.

- Supplements: Boost nutrition or tailor smoothies to fitness goals:
    - Green Power Powder: Nutrients of a veggie smoothie, without strong flavors.
    - Chia Seeds: Add protein, fiber, and nutrients with little taste impact.
    - Creatine: Support muscle growth and recovery.
    - Macha: Get a morning or afternoon caffeine boost.
    - Pre-workout: For extra energy if consumed ~20 min before exercise.
    - Disclaimer: Many supplements lack FDA evaluation – consult a doctor/nutritionist before use.

Pairings & Balance

Think of classic pairings you regularly see (strawberry-banana, chocolate-orange, carrot-orange, kale-apple-grape) and build from there. If including veggies, balance bitterness with sweet or acidic flavors.

- Smoothies are a great way to build confidence in your ability to create unique combinations – while some pairings work better than others, it's hard to go completely wrong (unless you're deep into the veggie/spice territory).

Other Tips

- Quantities: Per person, start with 1c frozen fruit, 1 banana, and 1c of liquid. If using fresh fruit, add ice to chill. Adjust water for consistency and start with 1/2t of any spice (if using).
- Bananas: Use fresh, or if you have too many ripe, peel and toss in a freezer bag.
- Coffee: Brew extra early in the week and refrigerate for easy smoothie additions.

Example pairings

Tropical Vanilla

Mango (frozen), Pineapple, Coconut Water, Banana, Vanilla Almond Milk, Vanilla Protein Powder, Ice

Peaches & Cream

Peaches (frozen), Banana, Unsweetened Vanilla Almond Milk, Cookies & Cream Protein Powder, Ice

Strawberry Orange Mocha

Orange Juice, Banana, Strawberries, Vanilla Almond Milk, Coffee, Chocolate Protein Powder, Cardamom or Mint

Vanilla Orange Banana 

Orange Juice, Vanilla Almond Milk, Banana, Vanilla Protein Powder, Ice

Orange Carrot 

Carrot Juice, Orange (juice or fresh, peeled), Ice

Fruit & Veggie 

Kale, Cucumber, Green Grapes, Apple, Pineapple, Orange Juice, Vanilla Protein Powder, Green Powder, Ice

Strawberry Banana Peanut Butter

Strawberry, Banana, Vanilla Almond Milk, Peanut Butter Protein Powder

Tropical Avocado 

Avocado (frozen), Mango, Pineapple, Banana, Coconut water, Vanilla Protein Powder, Green Powder

Mango Strawberry Vanilla 

Mango, Banana, Strawberry, Vanilla Yogurt, Vanilla Almond Milk, Vanilla Protein Powder, Cardamon

Chocolate Cherry Vanilla 

Cherries (frozen), Banana (frozen), Vanilla Almond Milk, Chocolate Protein Powder

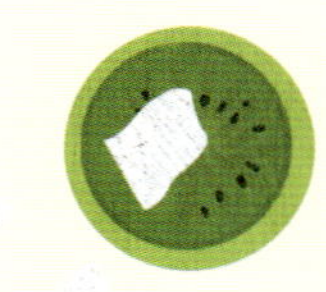

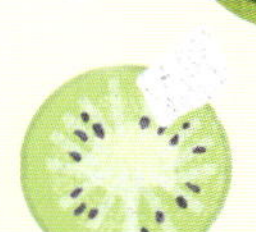

Açaí Bowl Framework

Think of this as a thick açaí-based smoothie served in a bowl, topped with fresh fruits, a touch of crunch, and a bit of sparkle.

2

Arrange as clusters in bowl on top of base with Sweet drizzled across top

Toppings

Granola/Nuts

- Granola
- Almond - sliced
- Cashew - crushed
- Macadamia - crushed
- Peanut Butter
- Sunflower
- Pumpkin Seed

Fresh Fruits

- Blackberry, Blueberry, Raspberry, Strawberry
- Banana
- Kiwi
- Mango
- Pineapple
- Pomegranate
- Avocado

Sweet

(if desired)

- Honey
- Guaraná Syrup
- Maple Syrup
- Mint
- Coconut Flakes
- Vanilla Extract
- Chocolate - chips/ shavings

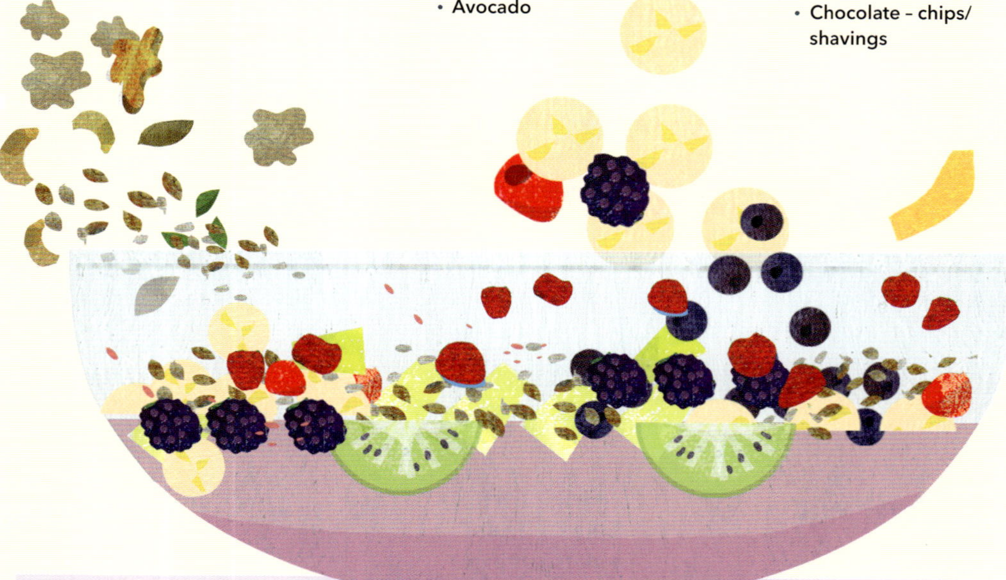

1

Blend Frozen Fruits first and only add as much Liquid as needed to purée

Base

Açaí

- Frozen Açaí Puree Pack (or Juice

Other Frozen Fruits

- Banana (recommended)
- Blackberry
- Blueberry
- Raspberry
- Strawberry
- Mango
- Pineapple

Liquid

- Coconut Milk/Cream
- Milk of your choice
- Juice
- Water
- Coconut Water
- Yogurt (or use as Topping)

Nutrition Boosts

(as desired)

- Protein Powder (Plain or Vanilla)
- Chia/Flaxseed
- Green Power Powder
- Creatine
- Maca
- Ashwagandha

Ingredients flow from easiest to pair to those inviting more creative consideration.

Tips on how to apply

Getting Started

All you need is açaí, which is easy to keep on hand with frozen packs available from Whole Foods to Wal-Mart. Everything else is optional or a pantry staple, with many ingredients overlapping with Smoothies.

Keeping it Healthy

While high in nutrients and anti-oxidants, fruits can quickly add up with natural sugars, so skip additional sweetener to keep it healthy.

- Calorie Mindfulness: Avocado, coconut and nuts while nutrient-dense, are calorie-heavy.
  - For Weight Loss: Keep portions moderate.
  - For Bulking: This is a great way to indulge while fueling up.

Pairings & Balance

The suggested ingredients all pair well together, so experimentation is encouraged – this is a dish that's hard to get wrong.

- Texture: Balance creamy (yogurt, nut butter, avocado) with crunchy (granola, cacao nibs, nuts).
- Contrast: Consider a pinch of salt or spices like cinnamon, cardamom, or ginger to add warmth and complexity.

Other Tips

- Prevent Melting: Chill bowls in advance so the base stays frozen longer.
- Social Spread: Set up ingredient stations so everyone can customize their bowl – just blend the Açaí base last to keep it frozen.
- Parfait: Layer in a tall glass with granola and yogurt to take on a new form.
- No Açaí?: Swap in other frozen berries for a similar base.

Example pairings

Classic

Base: Açaí, Banana (frozen), Coconut Water/Milk

Toppings: Strawberry, Blueberry, Granola, Honey

Builder

Base: Açaí, Banana (frozen), Vanilla Protein Powder, Chia Seeds, Plain Yogurt

Toppings: Almond, Mint

Tropical

Base: Açaí, Banana & Pineapple (frozen), Coconut Milk

Toppings: Mango, Granola, Macadamia, Guaraná/Honey

Peanut Butter

Base: Açaí, Banana (frozen), Milk, Protein Powder

Toppings: Apple/Pear, Granola, Peanut Butter, Chocolate (syrup or shavings)

Maple

Base: Açaí, Banana (frozen), Milk

Toppings: Blueberry, Granola, Maple Syrup

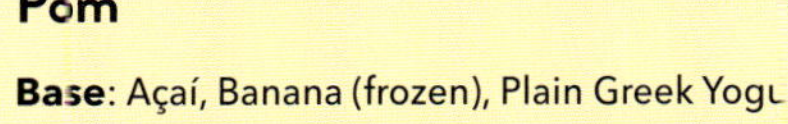

Pom

Base: Açaí, Banana (frozen), Plain Greek Yogurt

Toppings: Pomegranate Seed, Pistachio

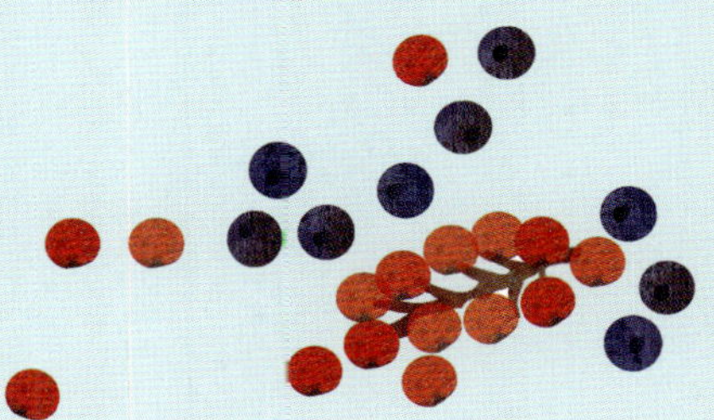

Overnight Oats Framework

Establish an evening wind-down ritual that sets you up for a healthy morning routine.

Combine oats, milk, and any boosts or accents you desire, then chill overnight so you wake up to a flavorful, ready-to-enjoy breakfast.

1 Core

Combine **Oats** with **Milk/Water** and any desired **Boosts**.

Oats

~1 cup

- Rolled Oats (not instant)

Milk/Water

(match Oat volume)

- Cow (Skim or 2%)
- Oat
- Almond
- Soy
- Coconut
- Water (for a lighter version)

Boosts

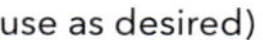

(use as desired)

- Yogurt
- Protein Powder (+ 0.25c Water/Milk per scoop)
- 0-1T Chia/Flaxseed
- Creatine

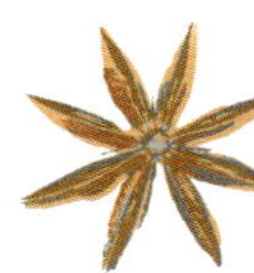

2 Accents

Add as desired

Fruits

(include selectively)

- Banana
- Fig, dried
- Apricot, dried
- Tangerine
- Pineapple
- Peach
- Apple
- Pomegranate

Nuts

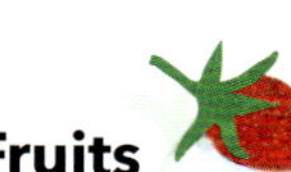

(optional; raw, roasted, or as nut butter)

- Pistachio
- Almond
- Peanut
- Cashew
- Hazelnut
- Macadamia
- Pecan
- Walnut

Sweets

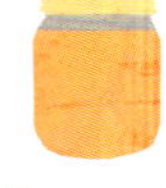

(1-2T, as desired)

- Honey
- Vanilla Syrup
- Maple Syrup
- Simple Syrup
- Lemon or Orange Marmalade
- Jam
- Nutella

Seasonings

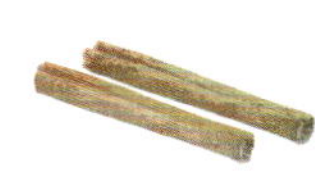

(include selectively)

- Salt (just a pinch)
- Vanilla Extract
- Lemon Zest
- Ginger Powder
- Cardamom, Cinnamon, Nutmeg, Star Anise
- Cayenne

3 Mix, cover, and refrigerate overnight

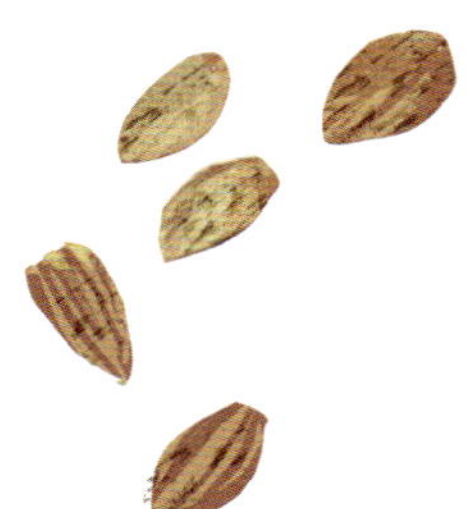

Serves 1-2.

Read from left to right as most essential to most optional, and from top to bottom as most recommended (lower listed items may require more consideration on pairing).

Tips on how to apply

Getting Started

All you need are oats - everything else is optional or a pantry staple. Many ingredients overlap with Salads and Smoothies, making it easy to repurpose.

Keeping it Healthy

Naturally nutrient-dense and high in fiber, so little modification is needed:

- Minimize Sweeteners: Use vanilla or cinnamon to enhance sweetness without extra calories (keep in mind syrups, jams and marmalades are essentially sugar).
- Boost Protein: Add a scoop of protein or yogurt for a more balanced, satiating meal.

Pairings & Balance

Use a smaller quantity of fruits than for Smoothies as oats already provide carbs (although oat's "net carbs" are low as most come from fiber).

- Texture: Contrast soft oats with crunchy toppings like nuts or crisp fruits.
- Contrast: Enhance sweet fruits with a pinch of salt or spice for intrigue.
- Brightness: A splash of lemon juice or tangy yogurt lifts flavors.
- Protein Powder: Vanilla is easiest to pair.

Other Tips

- Shelf Life: Stays good for 3+ days, so you can efficiently meal prep.
- Oat Varieties: Steel-cut oats require a quick pre-boil in milk/water - otherwise, this is a "no cook" meal.

Example pairings (always use Oats and Milk of choice)

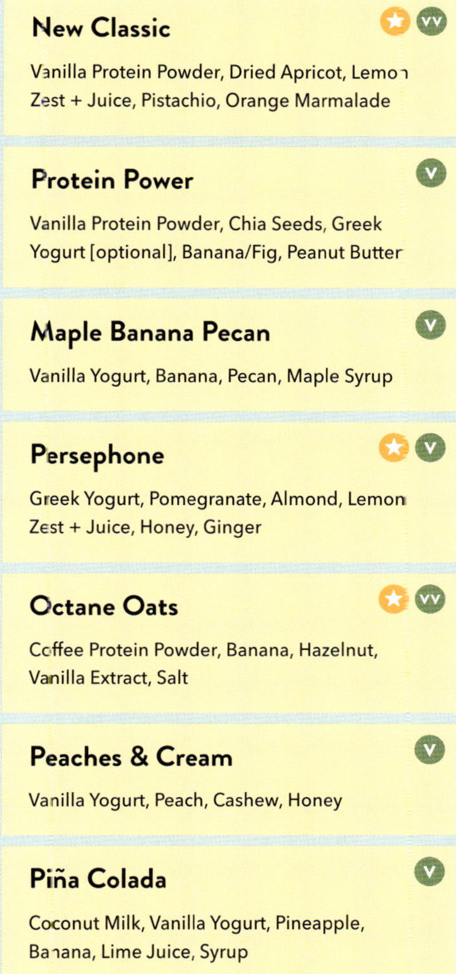

New Classic

Vanilla Protein Powder, Dried Apricot, Lemon Zest + Juice, Pistachio, Orange Marmalade

Protein Power

Vanilla Protein Powder, Chia Seeds, Greek Yogurt [optional], Banana/Fig, Peanut Butter

Maple Banana Pecan

Vanilla Yogurt, Banana, Pecan, Maple Syrup

Persephone

Greek Yogurt, Pomegranate, Almond, Lemon Zest + Juice, Honey, Ginger

Octane Oats

Coffee Protein Powder, Banana, Hazelnut, Vanilla Extract, Salt

Peaches & Cream

Vanilla Yogurt, Peach, Cashew, Honey

Piña Colada

Coconut Milk, Vanilla Yogurt, Pineapple, Banana, Lime Juice, Syrup

Scrambled Egg Framework

If you can throw together a salad, you can make scrambled eggs - just replace the bowl with a pan.

With eggs as your base, you can incorporate just about any veggie, protein, or seasoning. Simply sauté the ingredients briefly, then fold in beaten eggs.

1 **Oil:** 0.5-1T Olive Oil, Avocado Oil, or Butter — Heat in pan on medium heat (will also use in step 7)

2 **Onion:** 1/4 Yellow, White or Red Onion; 1 Shallot or Green
Garlic [optional]: 1-2 cloves - minced — Chop and add to pan to brown, ~3 min

3 **Veggies:** 0-2c: Bell Pepper, Fennel, Mushroom, Tomato, Broccoli, Artichoke Heart, Spinach, Kale, Arugula, Eggplant, Zucchini, Asparagus, Kimchi — Chop and sauté with Onion

4 **Proteins** [optional]: ~0.5c Cured Meat (Prosciutto, Pepperoni, Salami), Chicken, Sausage, Ham, Pancetta, Bacon, Chorizo, Salmon, Shrimp (shells removed), Tofu, or Black Bean — Chop as needed, add to Veggie mixture, and sauté ~2 min (adjust timing if using raw meats; reduce to 30 sec if using smoked salmon)

5 **Seasonings:** Salt & Pepper
Herbs: 0-1T Herbes de Provence, Tarragon, Basil, Oregano, or other dried Herb
Spices: 0-0.5T Paprika, Cumin, Chili Flakes, Soy Sauce — Season Veggie mixture as desired (will also add Salt & Pepper to egg mixture below)

6 **Dairy** [optional]:
0-1T Milk, Cream, Almond Milk, or Coconut Milk/Cream — If using, whisk with egg mixture in next step

7 **Egg:** 2-3 per person, whole or a mix of whole Eggs and Egg Whites — Whisk eggs with salt, pepper and Dairy (if using)
Add to Veggie/Protein mixture and stir until cooked (remove from heat just before fully set - residual heat will finish cooking)

8 **Cheese** [optional]: Parmesan, Feta, Goat, Ricotta, Cheddar, Monterey Jack, Mozzarella, Cottage, Fontina, Gruyère, Havarti, - grated/crumbled — Add to eggs when they are a couple minutes from being done cooking

9 **Garnish** [optional]: Caper, toasted Nut, sliced Avocado, or chopped Tomato
Fresh Herbs: Basil, Tarragon, Chives, Parsley, Cilantro, Dill - chopped
Sauce: Salsa/Pico de Gallo, Hot Sauce, Greek Yogurt, Sour Cream — Sprinkle on top/side and serve

Suggested quantities are per person.

Ingredients flow left to right from essential to optional, and top to bottom from easiest to pair to those needing more consideration.

Tips on how to apply

Getting Started

All you need are eggs - everything else is either a pantry staple or optional. Scrambled eggs are a great way to use any surplus veggies you have on hand, given their flexibility.

Keeping it Healthy

Limit the quantity of cheese to no more than a dusting and focus on lean proteins to keep this dish healthy.

Pairings & Balance

Eggs have a way of pulling things together in a way few other ingredients can, so it's hard to go wrong pairing any of the suggested ingredients together.

- Suggested Accompaniments: Toasted/grilled bread or lightly dressed greens, such as arugula.

Other Tips

- Technique: Stir constantly for small, creamy curds or stir occasionally for larger, fluffy curds.
- For Fluffier Eggs: Add a tiny splash of water instead of milk - it steams as the eggs cook, creating lighter curds.
- For Richer Eggs: Whisk in a small cube of butter before cooking, which melts and emulsifies for a silkier texture.
- Cast Iron: Use instead of nonstick pan for a more structured scramble - it helps develop slight browning.
- Reheating: Reheat scrambled eggs by warming gently on low heat - avoid microwaving on high to prevent rubbery texture.
- Alternative Eggs: Try duck (≈1.5 chicken eggs) or ostrich (≈24 eggs). Both offer a richer taste and creamier texture.

Example pairings

Protein Packed Scramble

Yellow Onion, Red Bell Pepper, Chicken Breast, Baby Spinach, Egg, Cottage Cheese

Garnish: Tarragon, Almond

Italian Sausage Mushroom Artichoke

Garlic, Caramelized Onion, Cremini, Marinated Artichoke Heart, Italian Sausage (Chicken/Pork), Egg, Parmesan

Garnish: Basil

Chorizo Avocado

Onion, Jalapeño, Tomato, Mexican Chorizo, Egg, Cotija Cheese

Garnish: Sliced Avocado, Cilantro, Hot Sauce

Smoked Salmon

Shallot, Cherry Tomato, Smoked Salmon, Egg, Goat Cheese

Garnish: Sliced Avocado, Chives +/- Dill, Lemon Zest

Shrimp Sesame Soy Sauce

Green Onion, Shitake, Eggs whisked with Soy Sauce and Sesame Oil, Shrimp

Garnish: Furikake or Toasted Sesame Seed

Tofu Scramble

Onion, Garlic, Bell Pepper, Cumin, Firm Tofu (crumbled, in place of Egg), Almond Milk, Vegan Cheese (Nutritional Yeast)

Garnish: Sliced Avocado

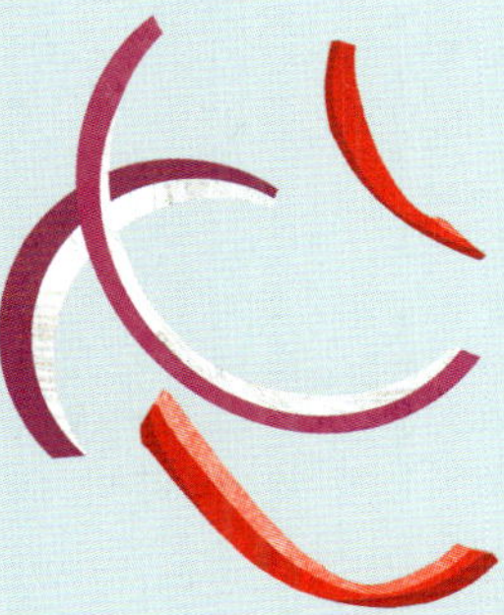

Omelet Framework

Think scrambled eggs, gently elevated –
a slightly refined technique creates a beautifully elegant dish.

While omelets use the similar ingredients to scrambled eggs, a touch of finesse transforms the outcome. Sauté fillings, cook eggs separately, then fold fillings into one half once set.

1 **Oil:** 0.5-1T Olive Oil, Butter, or Avocado Oil | Heat in pan on medium heat (will also use in step 7)

2 **Veggie**

Onion: 1/4 Yellow, White or Red Onion; 1 Shallot or Green

Garlic [optional]: 1-2 cloves - minced

Other Veggies: 0-1c Bell Pepper, Fennel, Celery, Mushroom, Tomato, Broccoli, Artichoke Heart, Spinach

| Chop and add to pan sequentially to soften

3 **Meat** [optional]: 0.25-0.5c Cured Meat (e.g., Prosciutto, Pepperoni, Salami), Chicken, Sausage, Ham, Pancetta, Bacon, Chorizo, Salmon, Shrimp (shells removed), Oyster, Calamari - chopped

| Add to Veggie mixture, and sauté ~2 min (adjust timing if using raw meats; reduce to 30 sec if using Smoked Salmon)

4 **Seasoning:** Salt & Pepper - to taste

Herbs: 0-1T Herbes de Provence, Tarragon, Basil, Oregano, or other dried Herb

| Season Veggie mixture to taste; cook briefly then remove from heat (will also add Salt & Pepper to egg mixture below)

5 **Dairy** [optional]: 1T Milk, Cream, Almond Milk, or Coconut Milk/Cream | If using, whisk with egg mixture in next step

6 **Egg:** 2-3 per person | Whisk eggs with Salt, Pepper and Dairy (if using)

7 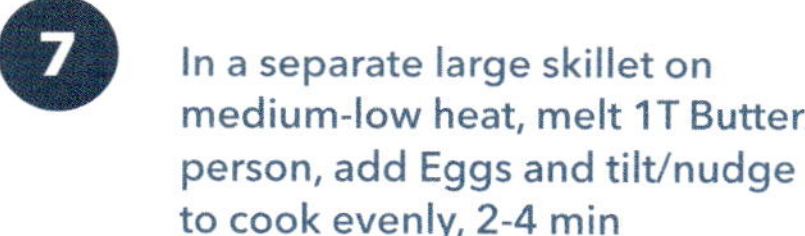
In a separate large skillet on medium-low heat, melt 1T Butter/person, add Eggs and tilt/nudge to cook evenly, 2-4 min

Add cooked fillings to half of omelet

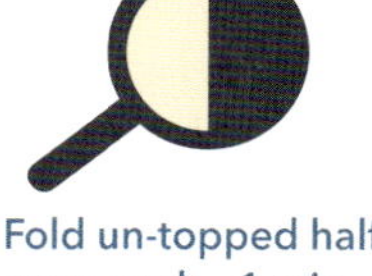
Fold un-topped half over, cook ~1 min

8 **Cheese** [optional]: Gruyère, Goat, Feta, Pecorino, Mozzarella, Havarti, Parmesan, or Cottage Cheese - grated/crumbled

| Sprinkle over Omelet (or include with cooked fillings)

9 **Garnish** [optional]:

Fresh Herbs: Chives, Tarragon, Parsley, Basil, Micro Greens, or Sage - chopped

Other: Butter, Caper, toasted Pine Nut, or chopped Tomato

| Sprinkle on top and serve

Suggested quantities are per person.

Ingredients flow from easiest to pair to those inviting more creative consideration.

Tips on how to apply

Getting Started

All you need are eggs - everything else is either a pantry staple or optional. Omelets are a great way to use any surplus veggies you have on hand, given their flexibility.

Keeping it Healthy

While naturally a healthy dish for being high protein and low fat, here's a few ways to maximize its healthiness, depending on your goals:

- Egg Whites: Use one whole egg + extra egg whites for a lighter omelet high in protein.
- Veggies: Load up on vegetables like spinach, bell pepper, or tomato to add volume and nutrients.
- Oil: Lean towards olive oil instead of butter.

Pairings & Balance

Eggs have a way of pulling things together in a way few other ingredients can, so it's hard to go wrong pairing any classic omelet ingredients together.

- Inspo: When you're in the mood to experiment, draw inspiration from other dishes - like our lasagna-inspired Tuscan Omelet.
- Suggested Accompaniments: Toasted/grilled bread, lightly dressed greens, fresh fruit.

Other Tips

- Cook Temperature: Cook eggs over medium-low heat for a soft, custardy texture; high heat will lead to overcooking.
- Style Variations: The framework suggests the simplest way to fold an omelet (in half) which is sometimes referred to as "diner-style" - a couple alternatives:
  - Thirds: Arrange ingredients in a row down the center and fold omelet in thirds for a more polished look.
  - French Style: Stir constantly while cooking, then roll it into a smooth, soft cylinder.
- Volume: You can create a "mega omelet" with up to 6 eggs in a single pan and divide into 2-3 servings when plating; if using >6 eggs, work in batches.
- Alternative Eggs: As with Scrambled Eggs, feel free to use duck (≈1.5 chicken eggs) or ostrich (≈24 eggs) for a more decadent version.

Example pairings

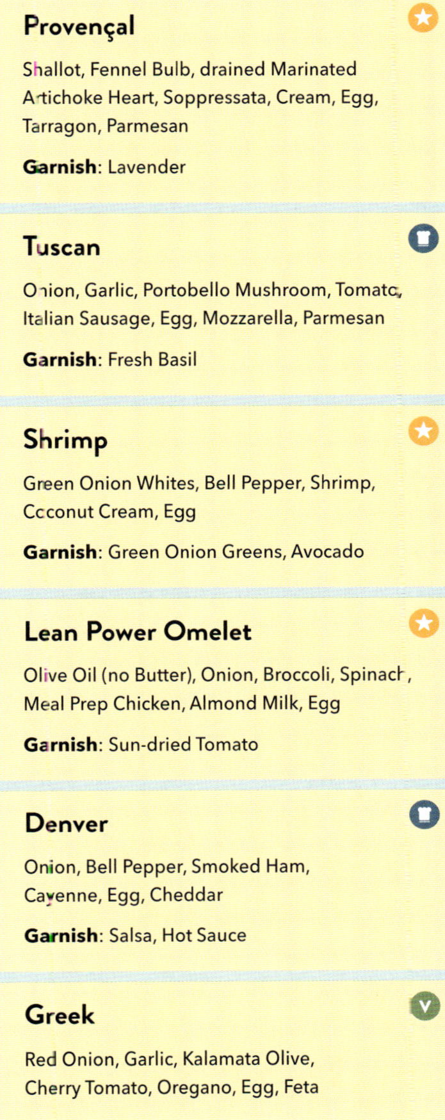

Provençal

Shallot, Fennel Bulb, drained Marinated Artichoke Heart, Soppressata, Cream, Egg, Tarragon, Parmesan

Garnish: Lavender

Tuscan

Onion, Garlic, Portobello Mushroom, Tomato, Italian Sausage, Egg, Mozzarella, Parmesan

Garnish: Fresh Basil

Shrimp

Green Onion Whites, Bell Pepper, Shrimp, Coconut Cream, Egg

Garnish: Green Onion Greens, Avocado

Lean Power Omelet

Olive Oil (no Butter), Onion, Broccoli, Spinach, Meal Prep Chicken, Almond Milk, Egg

Garnish: Sun-dried Tomato

Denver

Onion, Bell Pepper, Smoked Ham, Cayenne, Egg, Cheddar

Garnish: Salsa, Hot Sauce

Greek

Red Onion, Garlic, Kalamata Olive, Cherry Tomato, Oregano, Egg, Feta

Frittata Framework

Compose a sophisticated brunch dish that's uniquely yours – arguably easier than an omelet.

Frittatas are eggs at their most refined – elegant with light effort and capable of carrying heartier fillings than an omelet allows. Start with Italian flavors or follow your instincts around the Mediterranean, using what you have and finishing with fresh herbs for color and contrast.

1

Oil: 2T Olive Oil

Heat on medium in pan with sides at least 1-2" high

2

Onion

1/2 Yellow, White or Red Onion; 1-2 Shallot or Leek – chopped

Garlic: 0-4T cloves

Veggies

0-1c Tomato, Bell Pepper, Mushroom, Olive, Broccolini, Artichoke Heart, Spinach, Arugula, Pea, Parboiled Potato – chopped

Add Onions and sequence other Veggies based on firmness/required cook time and sauté 6-12 min

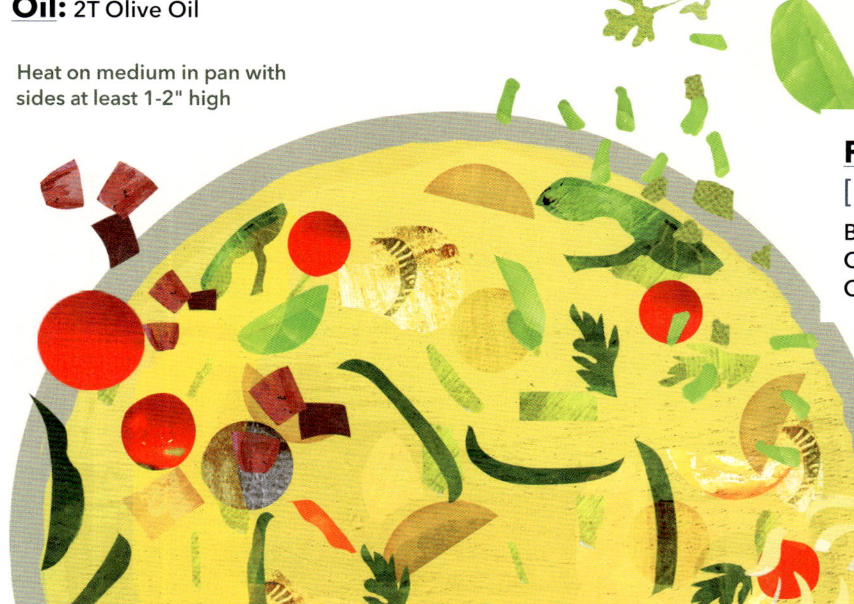

3

Protein

[optional]

0.25-0.75 lb Chicken, Sausage, Cured meat (e.g., Prosciutto, Pepperoni, Salami), Ham, Pancetta, Bacon, Chorizo, Shrimp (shells removed) – chopped

Add to Veggie mixture and sauté ~2 min (adjust timing if using raw meats)

4

Seasonings

Salt & Pepper – to taste

Herbs: 0-1T Oregano, Basil, Tarragon, Herbes de Provence, or other dried herb

Season Veggie mixture to taste

5

Egg: 2-3 per person without stirring

Whisk eggs and pour over Veggie mixture without stirring

6

Cheese

Parmesan, Pecorino, Mozzarella, Gruyère, Havarti, Feta, or Goat – grated/crumbled

Add on top and cook 8-12 min, until frittata is mostly set, with only a slight jiggle in the center and no visible runny egg on top

7

Fresh Herbs

[optional]

Basil, Tarragon, Oregano, Parsley, or Cilantro – chopped

Sprinkle on top and serve warm, room temp, or chilled

Suggested quantities are per person

Tips on how to apply

Getting Started

All you need are eggs, veggies, and ideally some cheese – everything else is either optional or a pantry staple.

Keeping it Healthy

Frittatas are naturally protein-rich. Load up on veggies for fiber and nutrients, opt for lean proteins, and use minimal cheese for a lighter dish.

Pairings & Balance

While slightly less versatile than omelets in terms of pairings, frittatas offer more flexibility to load up on fillings thanks to their sturdy structure. Start with Italian flavors, then explore outward across the Mediterranean for inspiration.

- Seasonal Themes: Incorporate roasted squash and kale in winter or peas and asparagus in spring.

Other Tips

- Pan Choice: While nonstick is easiest for stovetop-only cooking, use cast iron or another oven-safe pan if you plan to finish the frittata in the oven.
- Technique: Total cook time varies by ingredient volume and pan thickness – if the top remains undercooked, finish briefly under a broiler or in the oven.
- Texture: Keep the pan uncovered while cooking to avoid steaming and preserve a golden, gently crisp top.

Example pairings

Classic

Onion, Tomato, Egg, Parmesan

Chicken Power

Onion, Garlic, Chicken, Spinach, Egg, Lemon, Tarragon

Sausage

Onion, Tomato, Garlic, Sausage, Egg, Mozzarella, Basil

Shrimp

Leek or Green Onion, Garlic, Pistachios (roasted, crushed), Shrimp, Egg, Mascarpone or Parmesan, Coriander

Chicken Leek Mushroom

Leek, Garlic, Cremini, Chicken, Egg, Goat Cheese, Oregano

Veggie

Onion, Tomato, Bell Pepper, Artichoke Hearts, Broccoli, Egg, Parmesan, Basil

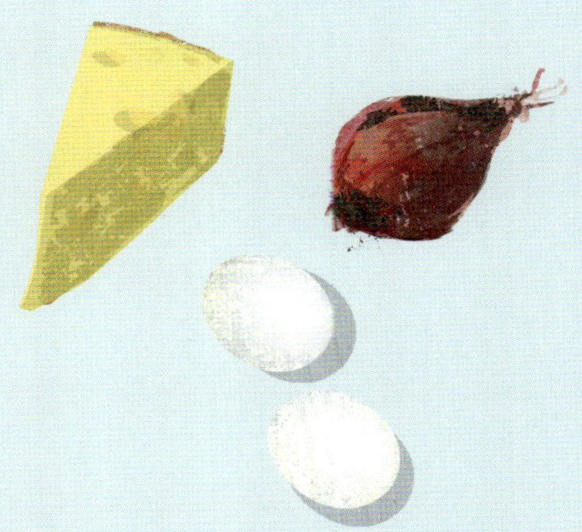

Shakshuka Framework

Delight your brunch guests with a showstopper that's surprisingly simple.

Shakshuka traces its roots to North Africa, and its spirit of simmered tomatoes with gently poached eggs spread across the Mediterranean in countless variations. Start with a spiced, aromatic veggie base, nestle in eggs, and let it come together gently on the stovetop.

Oil

2T Olive Oil, Avocado Oil, Butter, or 4 oz Bacon

Heat in large pan on medium-low heat

Onion

0-1 Yellow, White or Red Onion; or 1-2 Shallot or Leek - chopped

Veggies

0-3 Bell Pepper (Red, Green, Yellow), Eggplant, Mushroom, Zucchini, Carrot, Celery, Sweet Potato, or Roasted Pepper - chopped

Add Onions, soften, then add any other Veggies, if using and soften

Seasonings

Salt & Pepper - to taste

Tomato Paste: ~1T

Spices: 0.5-2T any mix of: Cumin, Coriander, Caraway, Paprika, Sumac, Ras-el-Hanout, Red Pepper Flakes, Allspice, Fennel, Cayenne, Turmeric, or Sichuan Pepper

Chili Sauce: 1-4T Harissa, Sambal, or Pilpelchuma

Garlic: 0-4 Cloves - minced

Add to Veggie mixture and season to taste

4

Tomato

~6 medium tomatoes (very ripe) or ~28 oz can - diced

Add to pan, simmer ~10 min to reduce liquid

[optional] add a splash of White Wine

5

Egg: ~6 eggs

Create wells in the sauce for each egg; crack eggs into the wells and simmer ~10 min

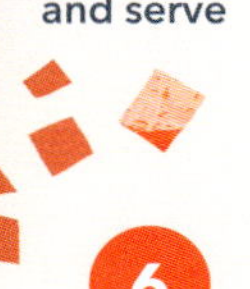

6

Meat/Seafood [optional]

Cured Meat: Merguez Sausage, Spanish Chorizo, Serrano Ham - sliced

Seafood: shelled Shrimp/ Scallop, cubed Ahi Tuna, Salmon

Nestle Meat into sauce as eggs begin to simmer; for Seafood, wait a few min after adding eggs to avoid overcooking

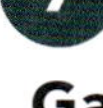

Garnish [optional]

Fresh Herbs: Parsley, Cilantro, Mint, Tarragon, Basil, Oregano - chopped

Citrus: Lemon/Lime Juice or Zest, Preserved Lemon

Cheese: Feta, Goat, Parmesan, Ricotta, Gruyère, Manchego - crumbled

Nut/Legume: Pine Nut, Almond, Pistachio, Chickpea - toasted

Other: Avocado, Olive, marinated Artichoke Heart - sliced

Distribute on top and serve

Serves 3-6. Accompany with toasted baguette or pita and optional salted plain yogurt.

Ingredients flow from easiest to pair tothose inviting more creative consideration.

Tips on how to apply

Getting Started

All you need are eggs, tomatoes and usually some chili sauce - everything else is either a pantry staple or optional.

Keeping it Healthy

This is a naturally healthy, high-nutrient dish that is difficult to make unhealthy, unless one were to load it up with butter and cheese - neither of which are necessary.

Pairings & Balance

Ingredients from all around the Mediterranean tend to pair fairly seamlessly - the main consideration is to avoid seasonings (herbs/spices) that clash or feel overwhelming in combination.

- Heat: Spicier versions particularly benefit from cooling garnishes like Feta or Yogurt.

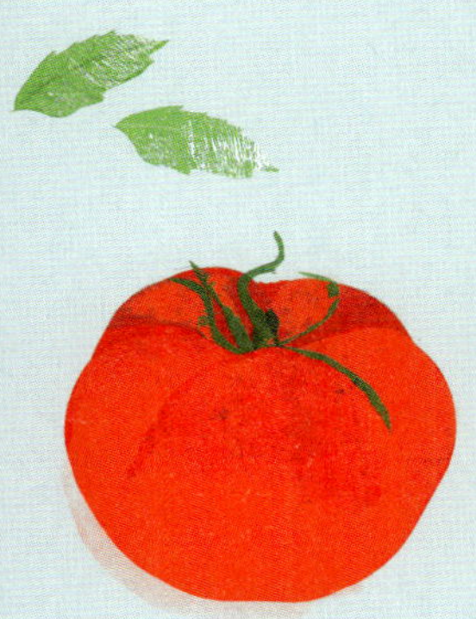

Other Tips

- Cooking the Eggs: If you like firm egg whites and jammy yolks, cover the pan while cooking.
  - For runnier yolks, leave uncovered and watch closely.
  - Stir the egg whites gently into the sauce as this helps them cook faster while keeping yolks intact.
- Batch Prep: Make extra sauce and store it - it reheats beautifully and works for pasta or grain bowls.
- Global Variations: While originating in North Africa, Shakshuka has an incredible journey of variations across geographies - some with key distinctions:
  - Algerian Hmiss: Roasted Red Pepper and Tomato (no Egg)
  - Algerian (eastern) Hmiss: above + Garlic
  - Algerian (northern) Hmiss: above + Egg and Caraway
  - Andalucian Huevos a la Flamenca: Spanish Chorizo, Serrano Ham
  - Balkan Sataraš: Bell Pepper, Tomato, Onion (no Egg)
  - Hungarian Lecsó: Bacon, Yellow Pepper, and of course: Paprika
  - Italian Uova in Purgatorio: Garlic, Eggplant, Parmesan
  - Tunisian Mechouia Salad: Cumin, Olive, Tuna, roasted Tomato and boiled Egg
  - Turkish Menemen: Green Bell Pepper, scrambled Egg

Example pairings

CookImprov Shakshuka 

Olive Oil, Yellow Onion, Red Bell Pepper, Garlic, Sambal, Tomato Paste, Ras-el-Hanout Tomato, Egg

Garnish: Tarragon, Lemon Wedge

Uova in Purgatorio (Eggs in Purgatory) 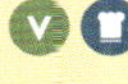

Olive Oil, Shallot, Red & Green Bell Pepper, Eggplant, Garlic, Tomato Paste, Red Pepper Flakes, Caraway, Tomato, Egg

Garnish: Parmesan, Basil, Lemon Juice

Andalucian Huevos a la Flamenca 

Olive Oil, Yellow Onion, Roasted Red Bell Pepper, Garlic, Paprika, Cumin, Coriander, Tomato Paste, Pea, Spanish Chorizo, Serrano Ham, Tomato, Egg

Garnish: Manchego, Parsley, Sumac

Seafood Shakshuka

Olive Oil, Green Onion, Red Bell Pepper, Garlic, Harissa, Coriander, Tomato, Tomato Paste, White Wine, Egg [optional], Shrimp and/or Scallop

Garnish: Feta, Cilantro, Lime; optional: Olive

French Shakshuka 

Olive Oil & Butter, Caramelized Leek or Onion, Cremini Mushroom, Garlic, Thyme, Bay Leaf, Peppercorn, Tomato, Tomato Paste, White Wine, Egg

Garnish: Gruyère, Tarragon

Hmiss (aka Algerian Salad/proto-Shakshuka) 

Roasted/seeded/peeled and chopped Red Pepper & Tomato - sautéed in Olive Oil and seasoned with Salt & Pepper; optional: Garlic

Bread Platforms

Sandwich

Avocado Toast

Bagel

Flatbread Wrap

Taco

Breakfast Burrito

Savory Crêpe

Sweet Crêpe

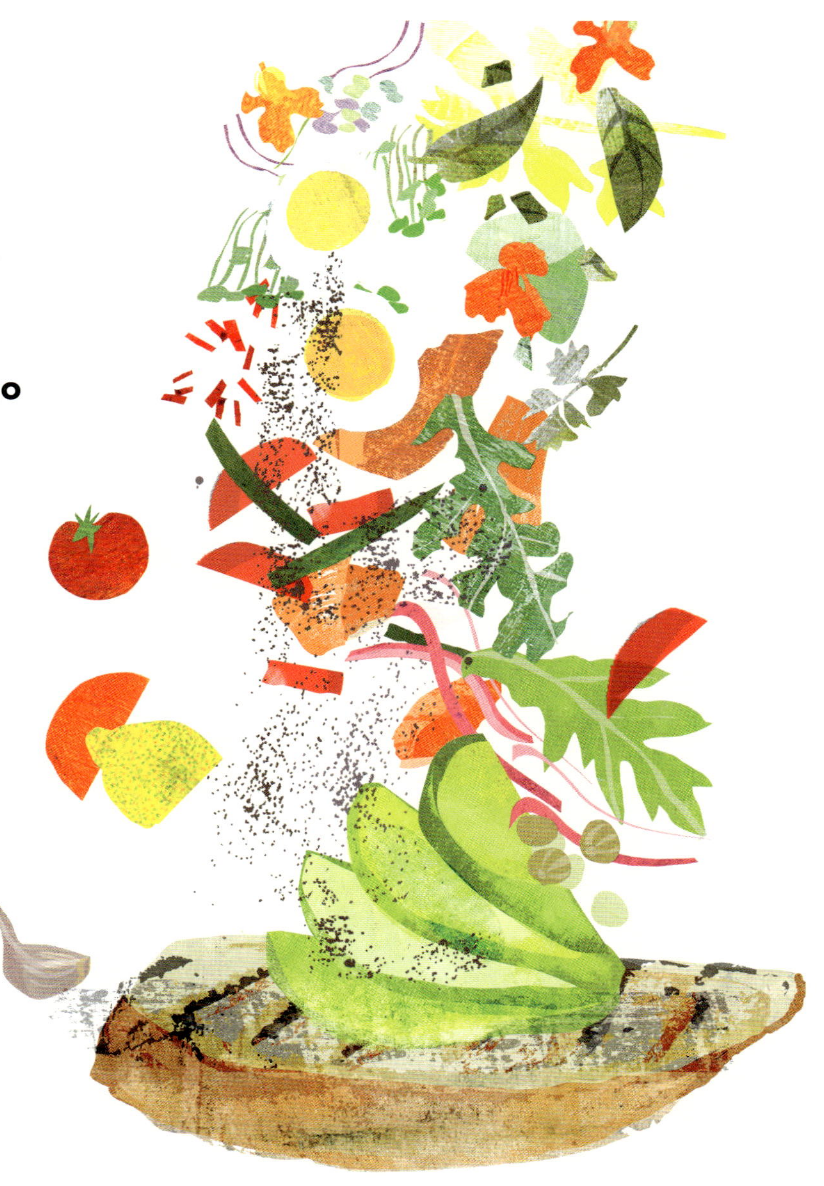

Bread takes countless forms, and the dishes built on top of it are even more varied. This chapter is all about closing the gap between what you make at home and what you'd find at a gourmet deli or hip brunch spot – and then going beyond.

These frameworks offer a unique mix of creative freedom and nutritional control. Because you can see and taste the impact of each component, they're a perfect training ground for improvisation, helping you build flavor intuition while aligning every bite with your nutritional/ fitness goals.

Sandwich Framework

The framework you never knew you always knew.

This framework brings structure to something deeply familiar. Start with crisped pread and finish with a satisfying press. Everything in between is optional: layer proteins, veggies, and pickles for contrast, then add seasoning or sauce to unify the flavors.

4 Complete sandwich, press, and enjoy!

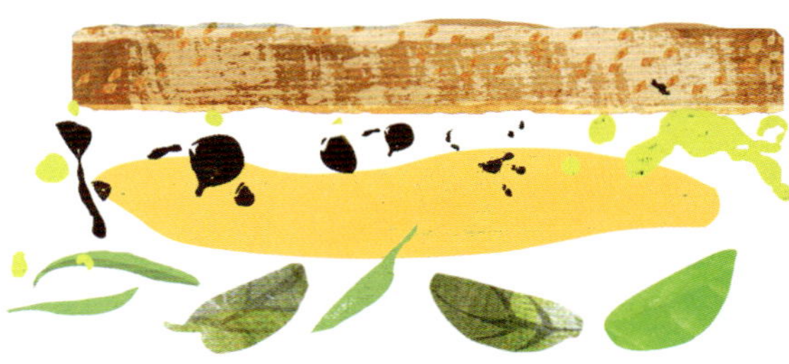

3 Layer toppings

Seasoning/Sauce [recommended]

- Drizzle: (Balsamic) Vinegar, Citrus Juice, and/or Olive Oil
- Spread: Mustard, Hummus, Olive Tapenade, or Chili Crisp
- Herbs: Basil, Cilantro, Tarragon, Parsley, Dill, Mint - fresh or dried

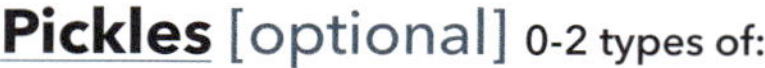

Pickles [optional] 0-2 types of:

- Cucumber, Roasted Red Pepper, Banana Pepper, Artichoke, Giardiniera (Italian pickled veggies), Carrot, Beet, Radish, Kimchi, Sauerkraut - sliced

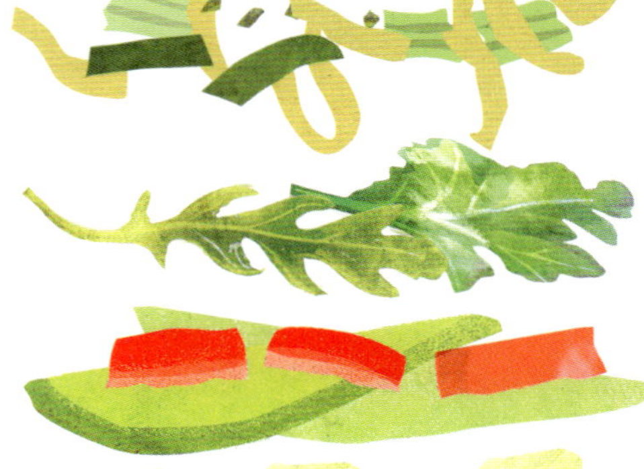

Veggies [optional] 0-4 types of:

- Leafy Greens: Lettuce, Arugula, Baby Spinach, Sprouts, Micro Greens
- Fresh (chose up to 3): Tomato, Onion, Pepper, Cucumber, Avocado - sliced
- Roasted: Brussels Sprout, Eggplant, Zucchini - sliced
- Fruit [occasional twist]: Apple, Pear, or Mango - sliced

Proteins [recommended] 0-2 types of:

- Deli Meat: Ham, Chicken, Beef, Turkey or Smoked Salmon
- Pre-cooked: Chicken, Beef, Shrimp, Sausage - warm or chilled
- Vegan: Tofu, Chickpea - roasted
- Egg: Over-easy, poached, or boiled and sliced - on its own or as an additional protein

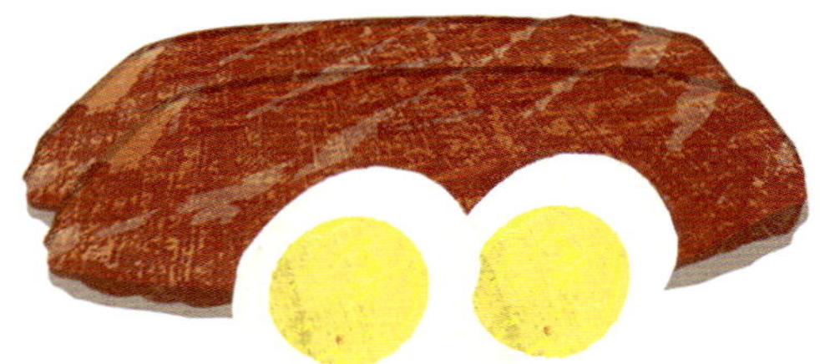

2 Add on top of bread mid-way through toasting to lightly melt

Cheese [optional] ~2 slices, any of:

- Cheddar, Gouda, Swiss, Provolone, Mozzarella, Parmesan, Pepper Jack, Havarti, Goat, or Feta

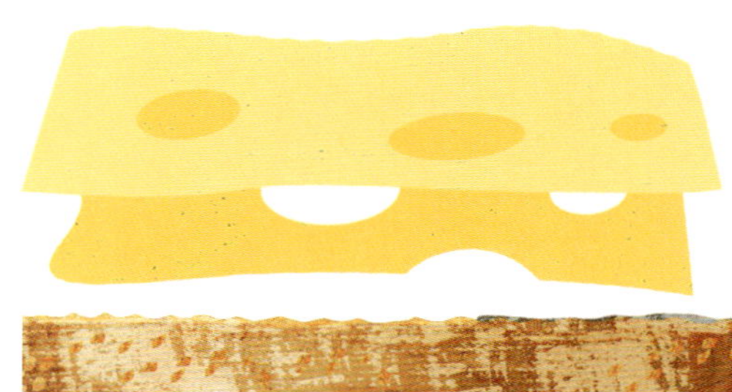

1 Lightly toast in toaster oven or on pan

Bread 2 slices of:

- Whole Wheat, Sourdough, Baguette, Focaccia, Ciabatta, or Brioche

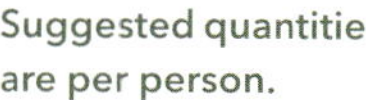

Suggested quantities are per person.

Within each category, ingredients flow from easiest to pair to those that invite more thoughtful matching.

Tips on how to apply

Getting Started

Many of the ingredients you'll already have in your pantry - to kickstart your sandwich game, pick up a couple deli meats and cheeses, which generally have a decent shelf life. Beyond that, the only critical perishable ingredient is bread.

Keeping it Healthy

- Meat: Deli meats (especially ham) can vary widely in fat content - look for options where the grams of protein outweigh the grams of fat.
- Cheese: Also vary widely in terms of healthiness. This framework prioritizes the healthier options - look for those with more Protein than Fat.
- Eggs: Boil or lightly fry eggs in olive oil to keep them healthy. Boiled egg whites are the leanest; it's generally worth keeping yolks for the added protein and nutrients.
- Bread: Cut thinner to reduce carbs, or use a lettuce wrap instead.

Pairings & Balance

Sandwiches are particularly flexible, so feel free to experiment or leverage combinations you've liked in other dishes.

Other Tips

- Toasting: While not required, has a big impact on flavor and texture.
- Press: Giving the sandwich a light press at the end has more benefits than you might expect.
- Onion: Use in moderation or consider sautéing to mellow taste.

Example pairings

New Classic

Whole Wheat, Smoked Gouda, Ham, Arugula, Tomato, Balsamic Vinegar, Olive Oil

Bistro Chicken

Thinly cross-sliced Baguette, Swiss, Meal Prep Chicken, Lettuce, Tomato, Red Onion, Tarragon, Dijon

New Orleans 

French Bread, Cajun-Seasoned Meal Prep Garlic Shrimp, Chives/Green Onion, Mayo, Mustard, Lemon, Salt & Pepper

Chicken Hummus Pita

Pita, Meal Prep Chicken, Tomato, Onion, Hummus, Tahini, Parsley

Modified Monsieur

Bread dripped in beaten Egg and grilled, Gruyère (or Gouda), Ham, Salt & Pepper

Mediterranean Veggie 

Ciabatta, Feta [optional], Cucumber, Tomato, Roasted Red Pepper, (pickled) Red Onion, Sunflower Seed, Hummus, Basil, Lemon Juice

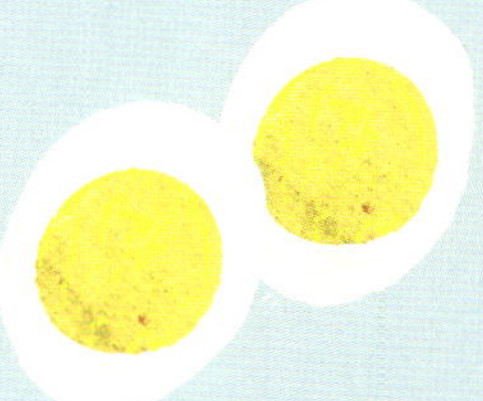

Avocado Toast Framework

Create the next cult-classic avocado toast – faster than standing in line.

This framework starts with crusty toast and seasoned avocado – from there, go minimalist or go wild. Add some veggies, a protein, or a sprinkling of herbs. Use the categories to build contrast and character or pick a theme and run with it.

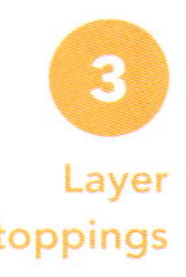

3 Layer toppings

Herbs [suggested]

- Fresh Cilantro, Basil, Tarragon, Parsley, Scallions, Dill, Microgreens, Edible Flowers, or other Herbs – chopped

Egg [optional]

- Sunny-side up, poached, scrambled, or hard-boiled and sliced

Meat or Cheese [optional]

- Meal Prep Chicken, Bacon, Meal Prep Shrimp – diced
- Smoked Salmon, Prosciutto, or seared Scallops
- Fresh Mozzarella, Burrata or Queso Fresco

Veggies 1-4 types of:

- Tomato, Bell Pepper – sliced
- (Red) Onion – fresh thinly sliced or pickled
- Arugula or other leafy greens
- Chili: Jalapeño, Banana, Anaheim – thinly sliced
- Capers or other pickled Veggies

2 Mash together or layer

Seasoning

- Salt & Pepper
- Spice [optional]: Paprika, Cayenne, Red Pepper Flakes
- Sauce [optional]: Pico de Gallo, Chimichurri, Pesto, Tahini, Harissa, Balsamic Glaze

Citrus Juice

- 1/2 Lime, Lemon, or 1/4 Orange

Avocado

- Ripe, mashed (skin and pit removed) or thinly sliced and fanned out

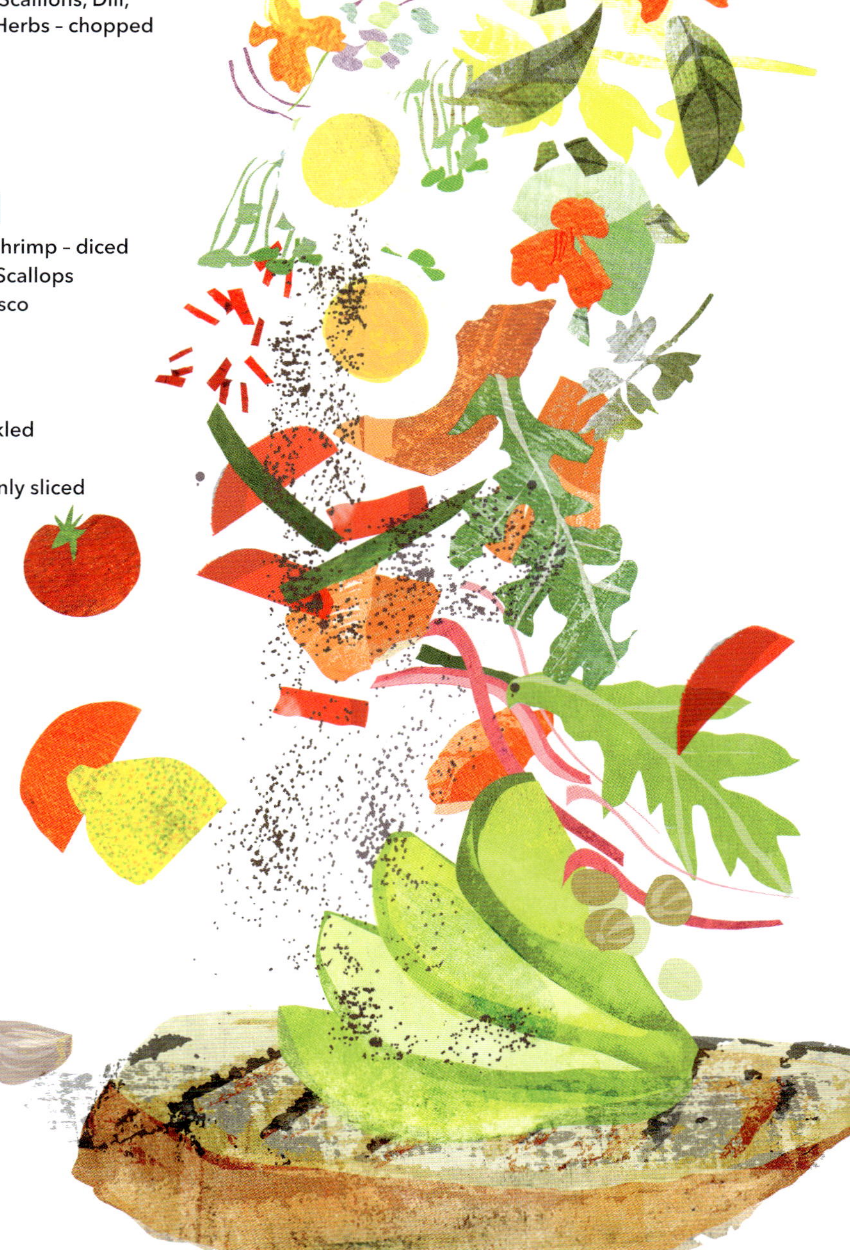

1 Drizzle in Oil and grill/toast

Bread

- Medium thick slice of sourdough, whole grain country bread, ciabatta - rubbed with Garlic if desired

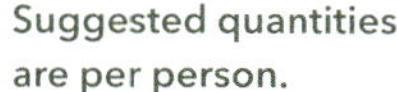

Suggested quantities are per person.

Within each category, ingredients flow from easiest to pair to those that invite more thoughtful matching.

Tips on how to apply

Getting Started

All you really need is quality fresh bread, ripe avocado, and citrus juice - everything else is optional or a kitchen staple.

Keeping it Healthy

- While not ideal for low-carb diets, this is a nutrient-dense meal packed with healthy fats, fiber and vitamins.

Pairings & Balance

Simplicity is key - avocado toast shines with just a few well-chosen toppings.

- Seasoning: Salt + a bit of pepper is often enough - if adding more, stick to just 1 additional seasoning to avoid overpowering the avocado.

Other Tips

- Toasting: Try grilling the bread for a charred, smoky depth.
- Social Spread: Prep ingredients ahead - toast the bread and mash the avocado with citrus and seasoning in advance - let guests assemble their own.
- Keep it Fresh: If preparing in advance, add citrus and cover mashed avocado with plastic wrap directly on surface to prevent browning.

Example pairings (use Avocado and bread of choice)

Classic

Lime, Paprika, Tomato, Arugula, Red Onion, Egg, Cilantro

Chicken

Lemon, Tomato, Pickled Onion, Meal Prep Chicken, Tarragon

ABLT

Lime, Cayenne, Butter Lettuce, Tomato, Bacon

Shrimp

Yuzu/Lime, Shichimi Togarashi, Meal Prep Shrimp, Sesame Seed

Burrata Balsamic

Garlic, Lemon, Arugula, Tomato, Basil, Burrata, Balsamic Glaze

Mediterranean

Garlic, Lemon, Tahini, Tomato, Red Onion, Caper, Parsley

Veggie

Lemon, Arugula, Tomato, Pickled Red Onion, Caper

Bagel Framework

Remix the sandwich – circular, schmear-forward, and layered with intention.

Beyond the bagel's toasty base, schmear and protein set the tone. Use a pre-made schmear or take a moment to customize, creating a spread that's simultaneously superior in taste and nutrition – then layer ingredients with contrast and character.

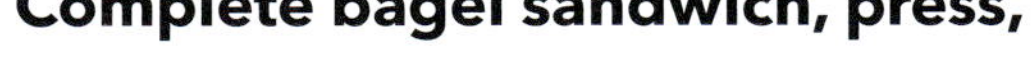

Complete bagel sandwich, press, and enjoy!

Sprinkle as desired

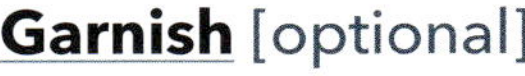

Garnish [optional]

- Herbs: Dill, Chives, Parsley, Basil, Tarragon, Cilantro, Mint, Rosemary, Perilla/Shiso – chopped
- Citrus: Lemon/Lime Wedge

Layer toppings

Pickles [sparingly] 0-2 types of:

- Caper, Red Onion, Gherkin, Olive, Roasted Red Pepper, Fennel, Jalapeño, Carrot, Daikon, Sauerkraut, Kimchi

Veggies [optional]

- Onion: Red Onion, Green Onion, Shallot, Fennel – very thinly sliced
- Fresh: Tomato, Avocado, Cucumber, Bell Pepper, Carrot, Radish - thinly sliced
- Leafy Greens: Arugula, Baby Spinach, Butter Lettuce, Microgreens, Sprouts

Proteins [optional]

- Crudo & Cured: Lox, Gravlax, Smoked Trout, Prosciutto, Salami, Bacon, Smoked Turkey, seared Ahi Tuna, Salmon Roe, Sardine
- Pre-cooked: Chicken, Beef, Tofu – sliced
- Egg: Over-easy, scrambled, or boiled and sliced – on its own or as an additional protein

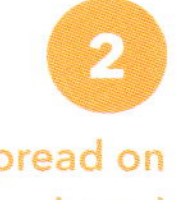

Spread on bagel

Schmear

- Cream Cheese, Greek Yogurt, Whipped Ricotta, Labneh, Mashed Avocado, Hummus, Mustard, Crème Fraîche, Olive Oil, Cheddar spread, Pâté

To customize: start with 4 parts cream cheese or Greek yogurt. Add ½ to 1 part Flavor Boost – taste, adjust, and riff as you go.

Flavor Boosts

- Herby: Dill, Chives, Parsley, Basil, Tarragon, Cilantro,
- Savory: Roasted Garlic, Caramelized Onion, Harissa, Smoked Paprika, Dijon, Green Onion
- Tangy & Bright: Lemon Zest/Juice, Lime Zest/Juice, Caper, Vinegar Reduction
- Sweet: Mashed Berries or Jam, Honey, Maple Syrup
- Umami: Sun-Dried Tomato, Pesto, Olive Tapenade
- Spicy: Harissa, Gochujang, Sriracha, Togarashi

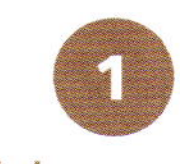

Lightly toast

Bagel

- Plain, Whole Wheat, Pumpernickel, Sesame, Poppy, Everything, Onion, Sourdough, Cinnamon Raisin

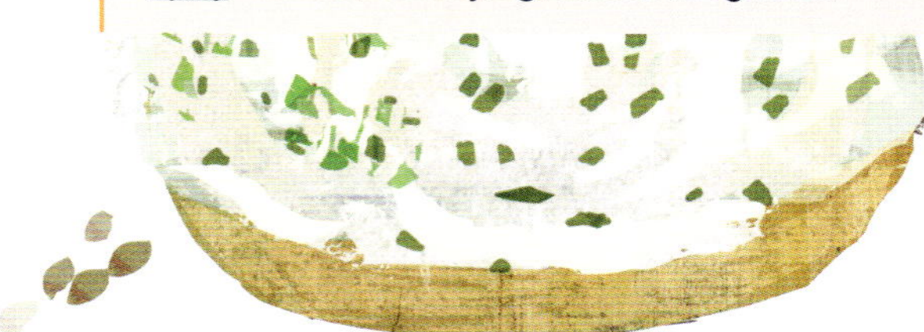

Suggested quantities are per person.

Within each category, ingredients flow from easiest to pair to those that invite more thoughtful matching.

Tips on how to apply

Getting Started

All you need are bagels and schmear - everything else is flexible. If you've built out a selection of herbs, sauces and pickled veggies, they'll be useful here.

Keeping it Healthy

- These can be dramatically lighter with a few tweaks: layer in plenty of fresh veggies, use cheese and meats as accents, and keep schmear to a thin layer.
- Cream Cheese Substitutes: Greek yogurt or labneh adds creaminess while keeping things bright and fresh.

Pairings & Balance

Bagel sandwiches are all about contrast - smooth and crunchy, rich and bright, herbaceous and tangy. Creamy schmears balance crisp veggies and acidic pickles, while herbs and citrus lift heavier elements like eggs, smoked fish, or cured meat.

Start by choosing your bagel flavor and build around it:

- Neutral bagels (plain, whole wheat) pair well with nearly any combo.
- Bold bagels (everything, onion) shine with eggs, sharp veggies, and fresh herbs.
- Sweet bagels (cinnamon raisin, blueberry) pair surprisingly well with salty or spicy elements - try soft cheese, chili flakes, or pickled onion.

Other Tips

- Schmear: Greek yogurt pairs beautifully with citrus and herbs; cream cheese carries richer, bolder flavors.
- Social Spread: For a group, create a bagel sandwich bar - set out sliced bagels, schmears, proteins, veggies, and pickles so everyone can build their own.
- Hotel Breakfast Hack: Free hotel breakfasts are often basic - flip that to an improv opportunity: toast a bagel, layer cream cheese, sausage, and scrambled eggs to craft a sandwich greater than the sum of its parts.

From Scratch

1. Combine 4c bread flour, 1T kosher salt, 2.25t yeast (1 packet), 2T Sweet (honey, barley malt syrup, molasses or maple syrup); add 1.5c warm water gradually and knead ~10 min; rest covered in refrigerator overnight.
   - [Optional] Mix in shredded Asiago/Cheddar, blueberries, or raisins.
2. Bring to room temp, divide into balls, and poke through center to shape rings.
3. Boil ~1 min in ~12c water with 4T Sweet.
   - [Optional] Brush with egg white and roll in toppings (poppy seed, sesame, onion flakes, garlic flakes, caraway, cumin, fennel).
4. Bake at 450°F (232°C) for ~18 min until golden.

Example pairings (use bagel of choice)

Lox & Lemon

Lemony Cream Cheese, Lox, Red Onion, Caper, Dill

Mediterranean Chicken

Hummus, Chicken, Tomato, Cucumber, Olive, Parsley

Bacon & Egg

Cream Cheese, Fried Egg, Bacon, Tomato, Arugula

Prosciutto & Fig

Whipped Ricotta with Fig Jam, Prosciutto, Arugula, Black Pepper

Banh Mi Bagel

Pâté Schmear, Pickled Carrot and Daikon, Cilantro, Mint, Chili Flakes

Egg & Herb

Chive Schmear, Scrambled Egg, Avocado, Arugula

Flatbread Wrap Framework

Wrap up distinct flavors with the framework that pulls them all together.

Start with a pliable flatbread and layer your elements for contrast: a protein, something fresh, something pickled, and perhaps a bit of crunch.

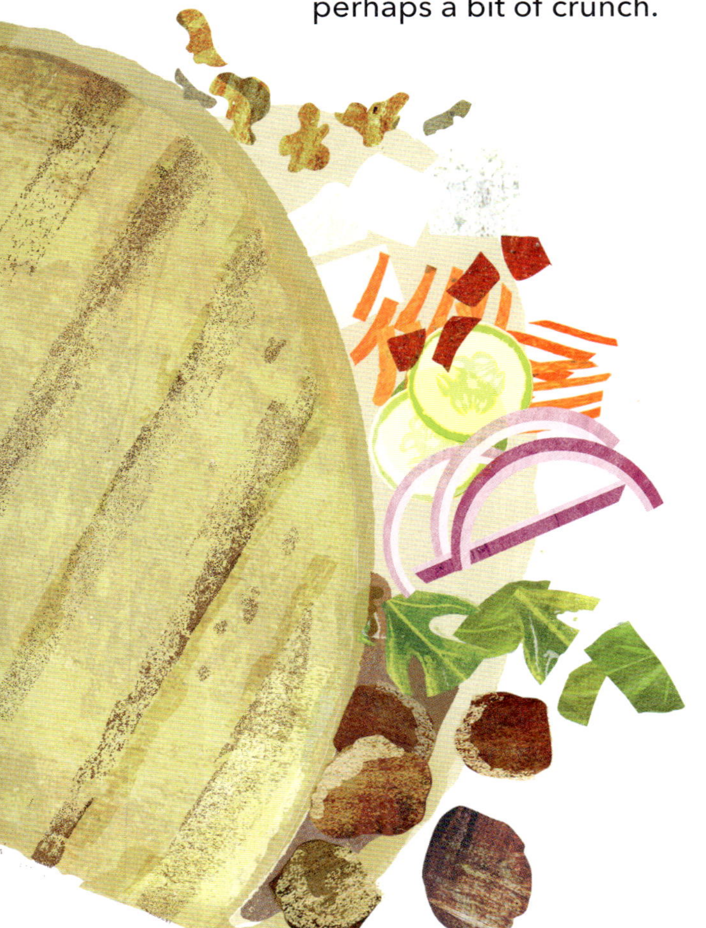

Nuts & Seeds [optional; toasted]

Pistachio, Walnut, Sesame Seed, Pine Nut, Almond

Cheeses [optional]

Feta, Goat, Halloumi, Ricotta, Mozzarella, Cheddar, Parmesan

Pickles [optional]

Red Onion, Olive (Black, Kalamata), Artichoke Heart, Beet, Cucumber, Banana Pepper, Giardiniera

Fresh Veggies [1-3 types]

Cucumber, Tomato, Bell Pepper, Avocado, Sprouts, Shredded Carrot, Ribboned Zucchini

Onions [thinly sliced]

Red Onion, Shallot, Green Onion, Yellow Onion, Fennel

Leafy Greens [chopped]

Arugula, Spinach, Herbs (Parsley, Mint, Cilantro), Leafy Green Mix, Baby Kale

Proteins [~0.5 lb; sautéed/roasted]

Chicken, Falafel, Roasted Chickpea, Beef strips, Ground Lamb, Salmon, Tofu, boiled Egg

Base Wrap [lightly toasted]

Pita, Lavash, Naan, Roti, Socca/Chickpea Flatbread, Tortilla

Build a Sauce

Simple Vinaigrette

Base
- Olive Oil
- 0.5T Vinegar

Flavor Boosts
- 0.5t Honey
- Garlic
- Basil

Citrus Vinaigrette

Base
- Olive Oil
- Lemon Juice

Flavor Boosts
- Garlic
- Basil
- Oregano
- Parsley

Yogurt-Based Sauce

Base
- Plain Yogurt
- Lemon Juice
- Olive Oil

Flavor Boosts
- Garlic
- Parsley
- Cumin

Tahini Dressing

Base
- Tahini
- Lemon Juice

Flavor Boosts
- Garlic
- Cumin
- Paprika
- Honey

Hummus Spread

Base
- Hummus (Cooked chickpeas, tahini, olive oil, garlic, lemon juice)

Flavor Boosts
- Paprika
- Roasted Red Pepper
- Garlic
- Cumin

Avocado Cream

Base
- Ripe Avocado
- Greek Yogurt
- Lime Juice
- Olive Oil

Flavor Boosts
- Garlic
- Cilantro

Aim for Vinegar/Citrus to be ~1/4 of Base volume; season to taste with Salt, Pepper, and other Seasonings, adjusting ~1t at a time.

Add optional Flavor Boosts to complement your wrap's theme.

Suggested quantities are per person.

Within each category, ingredients flow from easiest to pair to those that invite more thoughtful matching.

Tips on how to apply

Getting Started

As long as you have flatbread, you can make wraps with just about whatever you have on hand.

- Stocking: Long shelf life items like pickled veggies and nuts provide flexibility to elevate any fresh items and leftovers available.
- Sauces: Keep staples like tahini, yogurt, and lemon for easy, versatile sauce-making.

Keeping it Healthy

Small tweaks go a long way:

- Bread: Opt for whole-grain or lavash for added fiber and nutrients.
- Veggies: Fill at least half your wrap with fresh and pickled veggies for a nutrient boost.
- Cheese & Sauce: Use bold-flavored ingredients sparingly to keep calories in check while maximizing flavor.

Pairings & Balance

Flexibly pairable - tips to bring it all together:

- Texture: Combine smooth sauces with nuts or seeds for contrast.
- Brightness: Use lemon juice, vinegar, or pickled veggies to cut through rich proteins like beef or lamb.

Other Tips

- Sauce Building: A vinaigrette typically uses 3 parts olive oil to 1 part vinegar/lemon juice; reduce oil and increase acid for a lighter, brighter version.
  - Start with adding 1 minced garlic clove or 1t of mustard or fresh herbs (0.5t if dried) herbs - add more as desired; soon you'll have the intuition to skip measuring.
- Toasting: Lightly toast flatbreads to enhance flavor and keep them pliable.
- Assemble: Layer sauces and spreads first to help fillings stick and prevent dry bites. Limit filling to 1/3 of the flatbread to keep manageable.
- Wrapping: Use the easy wrap technique from the Breakfast Burrito framework or fold in half like taco.

Example pairings

Mediterranean Chicken Pita

Whole Wheat Pita, Grilled Chicken, Arugula, Red Onion, Cucumber, Cherry Tomato, Kalamata Olive, Feta, Pistachio

Sauce: Sweet Garlic-Lemon Yogurt (Greek Yogurt, Lemon Juice, Honey, Garlic)

Salmon

Lavash, Grilled Salmon, Arugula, Shallot, Cucumber, Carrot, Pickled Beets, Goat Cheese, Walnut

Sauce: Lemon-Herb-Yogurt (Greek Yogurt, Dill, Lemon Juice, Garlic)

BBQ Pork Pita

Pita, Meal Prep Pork (tossed in BBQ sauce), Cabbage, Bell Pepper, Pickled Red Onion, Cheddar

Sauce: Avocado Cream (Avocado, Lime Juice, Cilantro)

Spiced Lamb

Flatbread, Ground Lamb (seasoned with Cumin, Coriander, Paprika), Baby Spinach, Caramelized Onion, Cherry Tomato, Bell Pepper, Feta, Almond

Sauce: Tahini Dressing (Tahini, Lemon Juice, Garlic, Water)

Falafel

V

Pita, Falafel, Parsley, Pickled Red Onion, Cucumber, Cherry Tomato, Artichoke Heart, Feta, Pine Nut

Sauce: Garlic-Lemon-Yogurt (Greek Yogurt, Lemon Juice, Garlic)

Tofu & Pickled Veggie Naan

V

Naan, Tofu (Marinated with Garlic, Ginger, Turmeric, and Cumin), Baby Kale, Shredded Carrot, Pickled Red Onion, Cucumber, Cilantro, Cashew

Sauce: Yogurt-Curry Sauce (Greek Yogurt, Lemon Juice, Curry Powder, Garlic)

Taco Framework

Having mastered the sandwich, imagine tacos as dressing up in a fresh, vibrant new outfit.

Whether planning taco night or giving Meal Prep protein a fresh form, start with well-seasoned protein, then layer in veggies for contrast. Add grains or dairy if desired, then finish with any combination of seasonings/sauce.

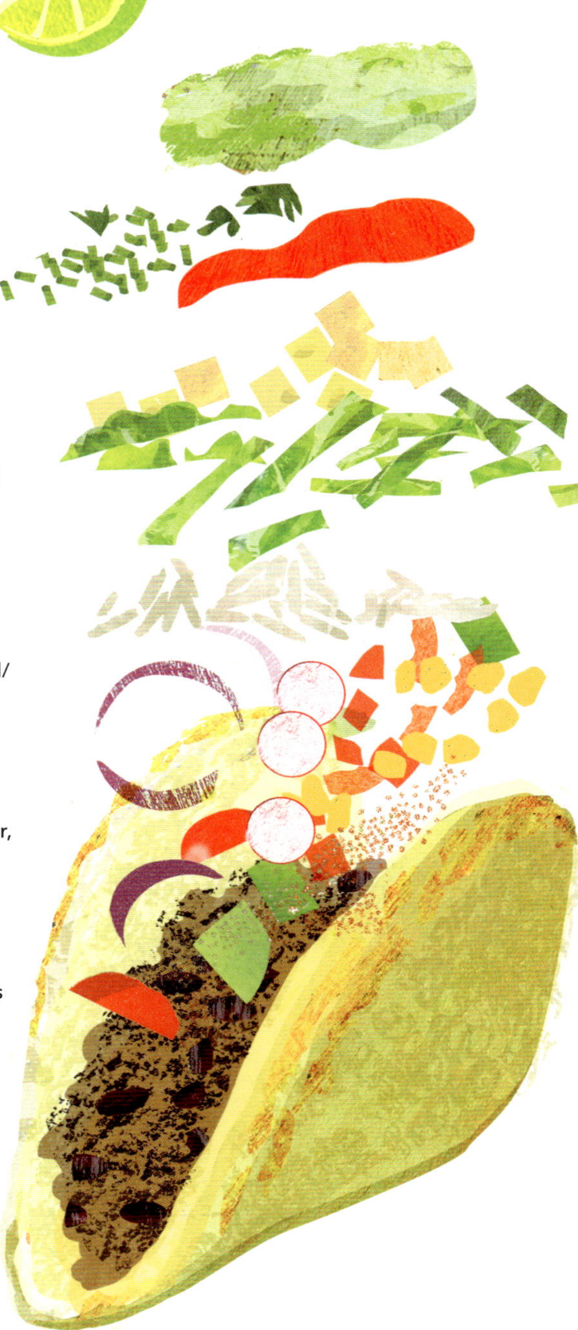

3

Drizzle, sprinkle, or squeeze as desired

Lime Wedge

Garnish [recommended]

- Sauce: Salsa, Guacamole, Chimichurri, Mole
- Herbs: Cilantro, Oregano, Parsley, Chives – chopped
- Hot Sauce: Your favorite variety

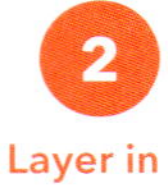

2

Layer in

Dairy [optional]

- Cheese: Queso Fresco, Cotija, Cheddar – diced or shredded
- Creamy: Greek Yogurt, Sour Sour Cream

Leafy Greens [optional]

- Lettuce, Cabbage, Arugula, Baby Spinach, Micro Greens – shredded

Grains [optional]

- Seasoned Rice or Quinoa – cooked with Spices and splash of Lime

Veggies [optional]

- Fresh: Tomato, Onion, Avocado, Pepper, Jicama, Cucumber, roasted/steamed Corn, Radish – diced/thinly sliced
- Pickled: Red Onion, Jalapeño, Pepper, Carrot, Radish – thinly sliced

Spices

- Cumin, Smoked Paprika, Chili Powder, Garlic Powder, Onion Powder, Coriander

Proteins [recommended]

- Pre-cooked: Chicken, Beef, Fish, Shrimp, Pork – chopped
- Crumble: Ground Beef, Mexican Chorizo, Tofu – sautéed with Spices
- Beans: Black or Refried – cooked and seasoned

1

Lightly toast on pan

Tortilla

- Corn, flour, whole wheat, or hard shell

Within each category, ingredients flow from easiest to pair to those that invite more thoughtful matching.

Tips on how to apply

Getting Started

All that's essential is taco tortillas.

- Stock long shelf life ingredients like dried beans, canned chipotles, pickled jalapeños, and hot sauce and keep limes and cilantro on hand to elevate your ad hoc taco game.

Keeping it Healthy

- Protein: Opt for grilled/seared/ roasted over deep-fried options.
- Veggies: Load up on fresh veggies like shredded cabbage, radish, and avocado for crunch and nutrition.
- Dairy: Use Greek yogurt as a base for crema-style sauces instead of sour cream.
- Beans: Can be a good source of protein/fiber (note: refried beans ≠ healthy).
- Grains: Consider skipping rice/ quinoa, as tortillas already provide carbs and this increases prep time.

Pairings & Balance

Tacos are flexible as you mix/match the suggested ingredients or adopt another cuisine into tacos (e.g., Korean Bulgogi Tacos), so feel free to experiment or leverage combinations you've liked in other dishes.

- Spicy Tacos: balance heat with something creamy, like avocado, crema, or cheese.
- Moisture: If using drier proteins (e.g., grilled chicken), add salsa/ sauce to keep it from feeling bland.

Other Tips

- Season Everything: from the protein to the slaw to the sauce, every layer should have flavor.
- Toasting: Enhance flavor and texture by lightly toasting tortillas/ taco shells.
- Meal Prep: Great use of Meal Prep Chicken/Beef, as it can take the form of an entirely new meal.

Example pairings (use tortilla of choice)

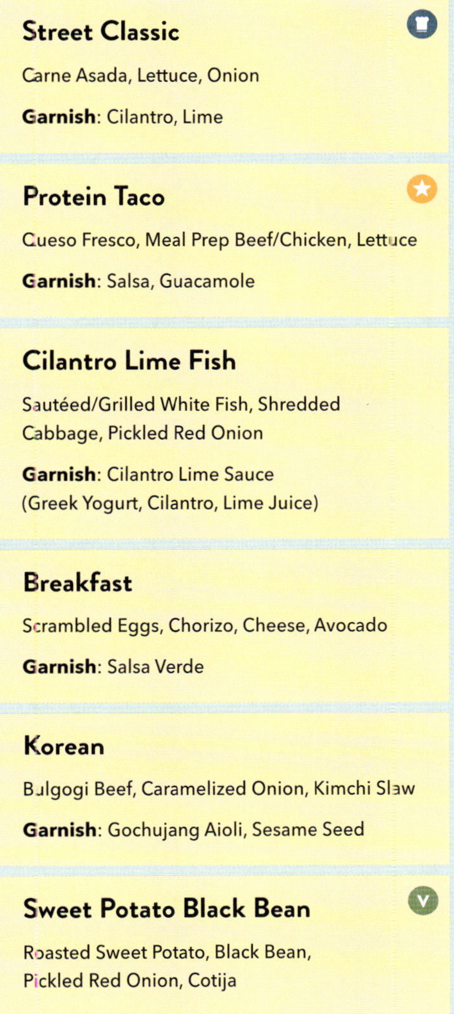

Street Classic

Carne Asada, Lettuce, Onion

Garnish: Cilantro, Lime

Protein Taco

Queso Fresco, Meal Prep Beef/Chicken, Lettuce

Garnish: Salsa, Guacamole

Cilantro Lime Fish

Sautéed/Grilled White Fish, Shredded Cabbage, Pickled Red Onion

Garnish: Cilantro Lime Sauce (Greek Yogurt, Cilantro, Lime Juice)

Breakfast

Scrambled Eggs, Chorizo, Cheese, Avocado

Garnish: Salsa Verde

Korean

Bulgogi Beef, Caramelized Onion, Kimchi Slaw

Garnish: Gochujang Aioli, Sesame Seed

Sweet Potato Black Bean

Roasted Sweet Potato, Black Bean, Pickled Red Onion, Cotija

Breakfast Burrito Framework

Reconceptualize Breakfast Burritos as scrambled eggs, wrapped in a tortilla, with potatoes or rice added for stability - served with a side of salsa.

Other than the tortilla, everything is optional: create a lean, protein- and veggie-forward wrap, or go full-comfort with gooey cheese and hearty fillings.

1 Scramble

[individually optional]

Onion

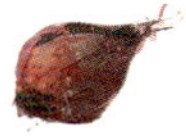

Yellow, Red, White - sliced

Other Veggies

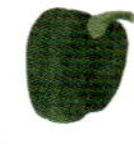

Bell Pepper, Tomato, Tomatillo, Mushroom, Spinach, Zucchini - chopped

Protein

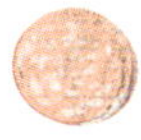

Sausage, Chicken, Bacon, Tofu, Chickpea

Egg

1 per Burrito

Cheese

Queso Fresco, Mexican Blend, Cheddar, Monterey Jack - shredded

Seasonings

Salt, Pepper, and desired Spices (e.g., Garlic, Paprika, Onion Powder, Oregano, Chili Powder, Cumin)

2 Prep Add-Ins

[optional]

Starch

- Rice: White, Brown
- Potato: Yucon, Red, Sweet

Herbs

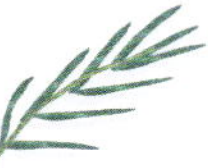

- Cilantro, Green Onion Greens, Parsley

Lime

- Slice in wedges to squeeze over Burritos

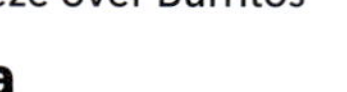

Salsa

Hot Sauce

Avocado

- Slice or prepare Guacamole

3 Assemble

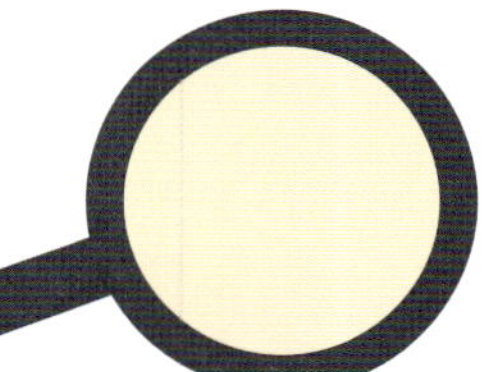

Briefly heat Tortilla in a dry pan

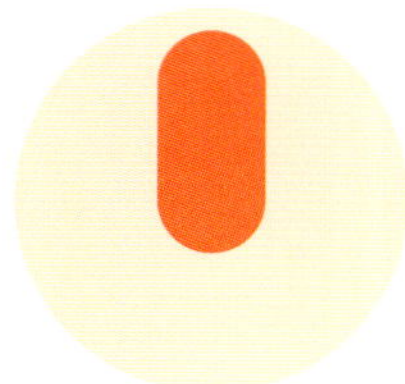

Lay Starch on burrito; layer scrambled Veggies, Protein, Herbs, Avocado

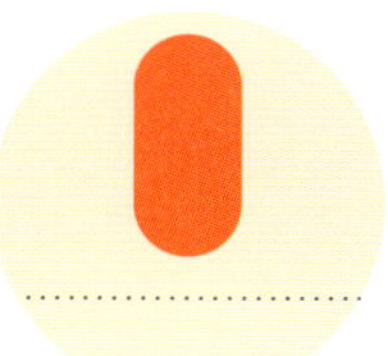

Fold up bottom edge

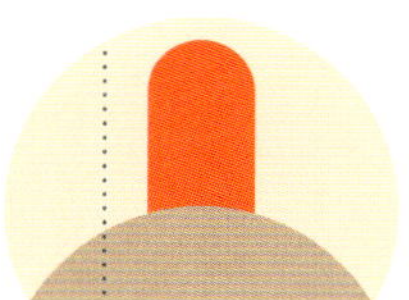

Fold in one side edge

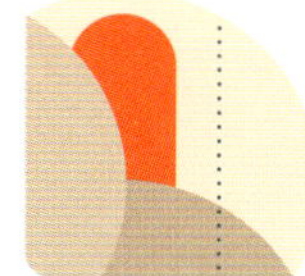

Fold in other side edge

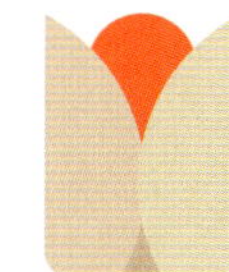

Add Salsa, Hot Sauce and Lime Juice or serve on side

Within each category, ingredients flow from easiest to pair to those that invite more thoughtful matching.

While not the traditional way to wrap a burrito, I find this to be the easiest.

Tips on how to apply

Getting Started

All you need are tortillas, eggs, and salsa – everything else is flexible or a pantry staple.

Keeping it Healthy

Use a lean meat, moderate cheese, and moderate rice/potatoes, to make this a reasonably healthy start to the day.

Pairings & Balance:

The flavors of suggested ingredients tend to go well with each other interchangeably – consider including something crunchy to add texture: diced & pan-fried potatoes, roasted chickpeas, or even tortilla chips.

Other Tips

- Salsa: Serve on the side (along with hot sauce and lime wedges) to avoid soggy burritos.
- Eggs: Go lighter with eggs than when making scrambled eggs, so there's a higher ratio of veggies and meat; 1 egg per burrito works well.
- Rice: Can be seasoned directly for additional flavor.

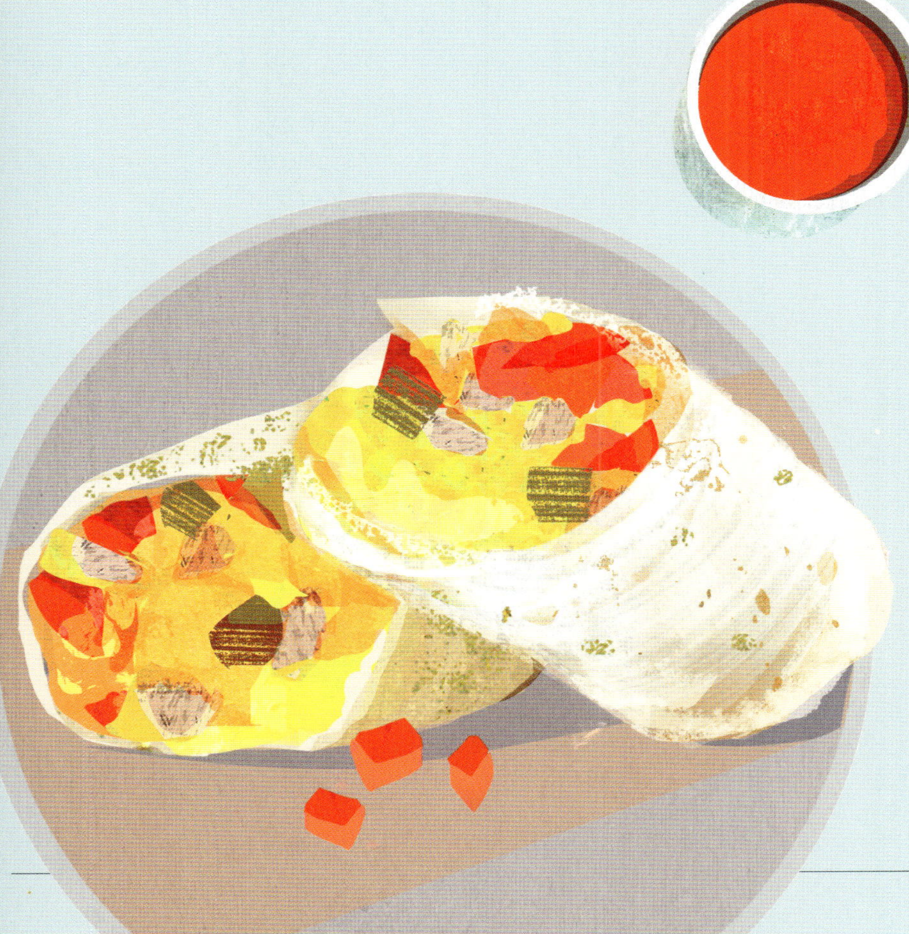

Example pairings

Classic Sausage

Pan-Fry: Yellow Onion, Sausage, Bell Pepper, Potato, Egg, Monterey Jack Cheese

Assemble: Rice, Salsa, Lime

Classic Chicken

Pan-Fry: Olive Oil, Onion, Red Bell Pepper, Tomato, Chicken, Egg, Queso Fresco

Assemble: Avocado, Cilantro, Pico de Gallo, Lime

Tuscan

Pan-Fry: Olive Oil, Garlic, Onion, Red Bell Pepper, Tomato, Italian Sausage, Egg, Pecorino

Assemble: Rice, Avocado, Cilantro, Pico de Gallo, Lime

Bacon Potato

Pan-Fry: Bacon, Potato;
Remove then add: Onion, Bell Pepper, Egg, Cheddar

Assemble: Rice, Avocado, Cilantro, Red Salsa

Variation: Substitute Bacon with Chorizo (and add Neutral Oil)

Vegan

Start with Tofu Scramble (from Scrambled Eggs Framework), add to Burrito with Rice, Beans, Avocado and Salsa.

Tofu Scramble: Onion, Garlic, Bell Pepper, Cumin, Firm Tofu (crumbled, in place of eggs), (Almond) Milk, Nutritional Yeast

Chilaquiles

Pan-Fry: Garlic, Onion, Tomatillo or Tomato, Jalapeño, then add a bit of Stock

Mix in: Queso Fresco + lightly fried Tortilla Chips

Assemble: Fried Egg, Avocado, Cilantro, Lime; optional: Shredded Chicken/Beef or Beans

Savory Crêpe Framework

Perfect the crêpe batter – then freestyle the savory filling.

With so many directions to take a crêpe, first decide if you'll be cooking an egg into the crêpe galette-style or whether you'll roll or quarter it. You can make the batter for savory crêpes, and mid-way through add a pinch of sugar, transitioning it to your dessert course (see next framework).

1 Whisk/Blend Batter

Flour 2/3c

Milk 1c + 2T (Whole, 2%, Almond, or Coconut)

Egg 2

Butter 2T - melted

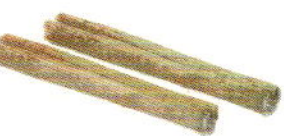

Salt Pinch

Seasoning/Herbs [optional] ~0.5T

Water Add in 1T increments if needed to thin (may only know after 1st attempt)

3 Make Shells

- Per Shell: Heat 0.5t Butter in pan on medium
- Pour ~2T batter into Butter on side of pan
- Tilt & swirl pan to spread batter into disc; flip after 1 min

4 Fill & Fold

- Cook for another 30 sec
- Remove from heat, keep warm while creating other crêpes or fill with any Sauce, Cheese, Meat, Veggies
- Roll or fold into quarters
- Garnish as desired

OR

Fill, Galette-style

- Crack Egg into center of shell
- Spread Egg whites, keeping yolk intact; cook ~30 sec
- Top sides with any Veggies, Meat or Cheese
- Fold in sides of shell to create square crêpe with yolk in center
- Garnish and Sauce as desired

2 Prep Filling

[individually optional]

Meats & Veggies Chop, season, and sauté (as needed)

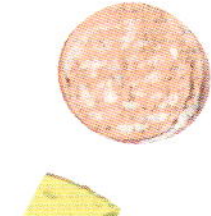

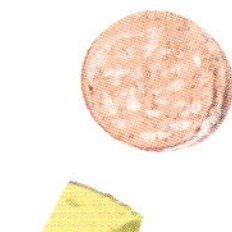

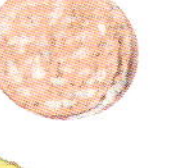

Cheeses Grate

Sauce & Garnish Prep and station

Roll

Quarter

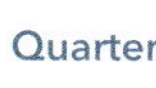

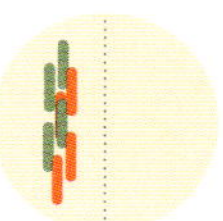

Galette

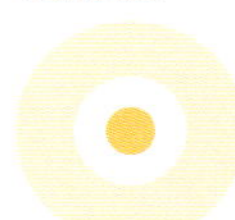

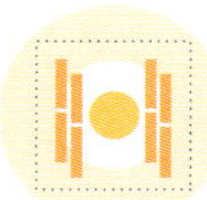

Suggested Ingredients

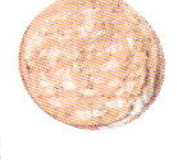

Meats

- Ham, Smoked Salmon, Prosciutto, Salami - sliced
- Pre-cooked: Chicken, Beef, Shrimp, Sausage, Ground Lamb

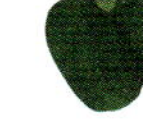

Veggies

- Onion: 0-1 Brown, Shallot, Green, Leek, Fennel - thinly sliced and/or caramelized
- Sautéed: 0-3 of Mushroom, Tomato, Bell Pepper, Zucchini, Eggplant
- Cucumber, Avocado - sliced
- Leafy Greens: Arugula, Spinach, Baby Kale
- Pickled: 0-1 Artichoke, Caper, Red Onion, Olive

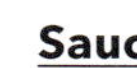

Cheeses

Béchamel, Mustard, Pesto, Tomato Sauce, Romesco, Greek Yogurt, Crème Fraîche, Sour Cream, Boursin, Tapenade

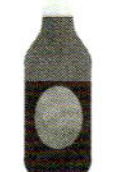

Sauce

Béchamel, Mustard, Pesto, Tomato Sauce, Romesco, Greek Yogurt, Crème Fraîche, Sour Cream, Boursin, Tapenade, Soy Sauce, Hoisin

Garnish

- Seasoning: Garlic, Fennel Seed, Black Pepper, Chili Flake, Lemon Zest
- Herbs: Chives, Tarragon, Parsley, Basil, Oregano/Marjoram, Thyme, Herbes de Provence - chopped
- Nuts: Almond, Walnut, Pine Nut, Pistachio - toasted, crushed

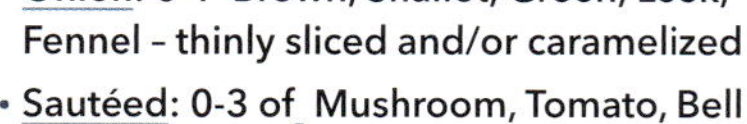

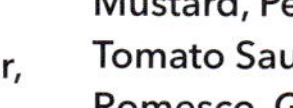

Creates 10-12 Crêpes. Serves 2-6.

Within each category, ingredients flow from easiest to pair to those that invite more thoughtful matching.

Tips on how to apply

Getting Started

All you really need are ingredients for crêpe batter and probably some cheese – everything else is flexible.

- Pan: Use a pan with low edges – no specialty crêpe pan required; key options:
    - Nonstick: Easiest to use, ideal for beginners.
    - Cast Iron: Traditional; enhances texture and browning, requires seasoning, heavier to handle and swirl.
    - Carbon Steel: Balances non-stick ease and cast-iron texture enhancement.
    - Electric Crêpe Maker: Useful if making high volumes or sans stovetop.
- Tools: Spatula (doesn't need to be crêpe-specific); optional: crêpe spreader.

Keeping it Healthy

Use cheese sparingly to keep crêpes light – boost nutrition and flavor by generously including veggies, leafy greens, and herbs.

Pairings & Balance

Classic crêpe fillings harmonize effortlessly. If exploring fusion flavors (like the Hoisin Chicken example) plan your combinations intentionally, aiming for balanced textures and complementary tastes.

Other Tips

- Buckwheat Variation: For a more distinct flavor, substitute up to 100% of flour with buckwheat flour, replacing an equal proportion of milk with water; buckwheat is trickier to handle, so try starting with a 50% blend.
- Gluten Free: Use almond flour in place of standard flour.
- Coconut Milk: If using canned, skim off the cream first, or plan to thin it with water for the right consistency – it's delectable.
- Batter Swirl: Lift the pan slightly off the heat when swirling batter to evenly coat without scorching or uneven thickness.
- Batter Consistency: Aim for thin batter, roughly the consistency of heavy cream, to achieve delicate crêpes.
- First Attempts: While early crêpes might not look perfect, they will taste delicious.
- Advance Prep: You can make the batter or crêpe shells a day in advance and refrigerate – doing so actually enhances the batter (particularly for buckwheat).

Example pairings (use tortilla of choice)

Classic Ham & Cheese

Ham, Gruyère or Swiss Cheese; optional: Honey Dijon Mustard

Garnish: Chives or Green Onion Greens

Chicken & Mushroom

Chicken Breast, Gruyère or Swiss, Shallot, Mushroom; optional: Béchamel

Garnish: Herbes de Provence

Tapa Style Garlic Shrimp

Garlic sautéed Shrimp with Olive Oil, Caramelized Shallot, Roasted Red Pepper, Paprika

Garnish: Parsley

Hoisin Chicken & Shiitake

Garlic-Ginger sautéed Chicken in Sesame Oil, Green Onion, Shiitake, Hoisin; optional: Sriracha

Garnish: Cilantro, Sesame Seed

Smoked Salmon & Caviar

Smoked Salmon, Salmon Roe, Crème Fraîche; optional: Shallot

Garnish: Chives

Ratatouille Crêpe

Caramelized Yellow Onion, Eggplant/Zucchini, Tomato, Bell Pepper, Garlic, Fennel Seed; optional: Fontina, Chicken

Garnish: Basil, Thyme, and/or Parsley

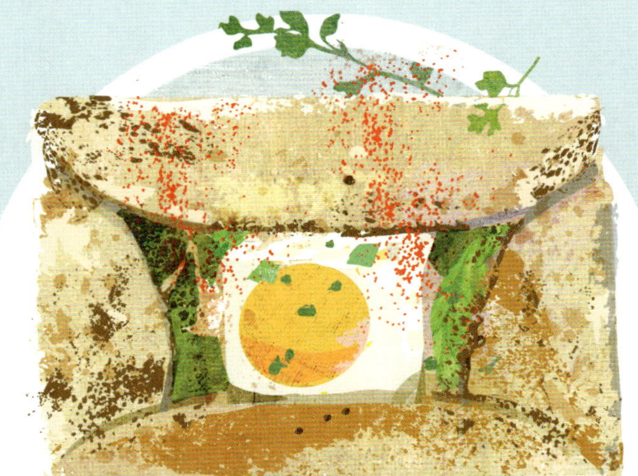

Sweet Crêpe Framework

Flip your crêpe-making skills to their sweeter side.

While Banana Nutella is a classic for a reason, these can be filled with endless com-binations of fruit, sweet sauces, dairy, nuts, and spices - even turning dessert into something surprisingly whole-some with the right balance.

1 Whisk/Blend Batter

Use Savory Crepe batter (p66) plus:

Sugar

1T Granulated, Powdered, or Brown

Optional:

- Liqueur: 1-2T Grand Marnier, Cointreau, Amaretto, Brandy or Calvados
- Powder: 2-4T Cocoa Powder, Matcha Powder, Cinnamon
- Extract: 0.5-1t Vanilla or Almond

2 Prep Filling

Fruit

Slice, mash, and/or cook if desired

Sauce, Dairy, Garnish

Prep and station

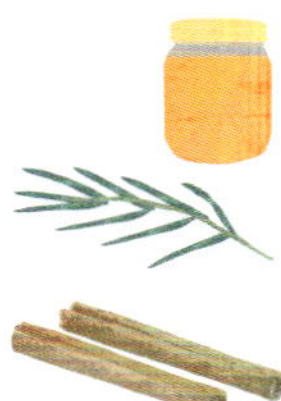

Make Shells

- Per shell: Heat 0.5t Butter in pan on medium
- Pour ~2T batter into Butter on side of pan
- Tilt & swirl pan to spread batter into disc
- Flip after 1 min
- Cook for another 30 sec

Fill & Fold

- Remove from heat, keep warm while creating other Crêpes or fill with any Sauce, Dairy, Fruit
- Roll or Quarter
- Garnish as desired

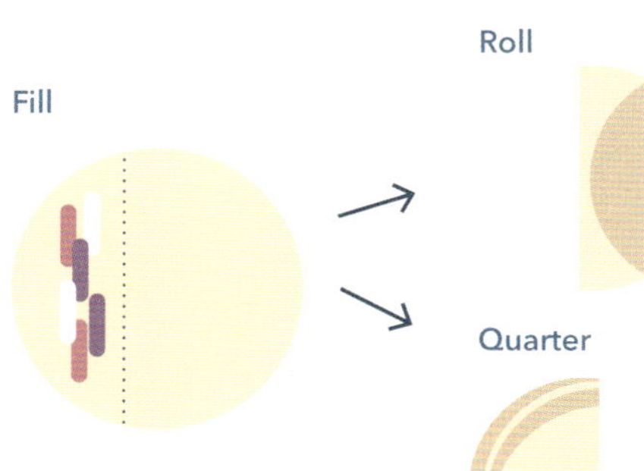

Suggested Ingredients

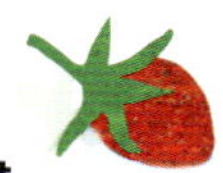

Fruit

0-3 of: Banana, Strawberry, Raspberry, Blueberry, Blackberry, Peach, Pear, Apple, Apricot, Pineapple, Guava, Cherry

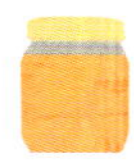

Sauce

Nutella (Chocolate Spread), Greek Yogurt (Flavored or Plain), Fruit Jam, Marmalade, Dulce de Leche, Chocolate Sauce, Salted Caramel, Custard

Dairy

- Cheese: Ricotta, Mascarpone, Cottage or Cream Cheese
- Cream: Whipped (optionally with Vanilla or Citrus Zest)

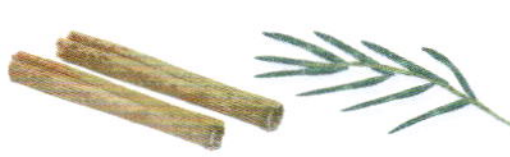

Garnish

- Sweet: Powdered Sugar, Maple Syrup, Honey
- Nuts: Hazelnut, Almond, Pistachio, Walnut, Pine Nut - toasted, crushed
- Spices & Seasonings: Citrus Zest, Cinnamon, Vanilla Bean, Nutmeg, Clove, Star Anise, Toasted Coconut Flakes, Cocoa Powder, Matcha Powder, Mint, Tarragon, Basil

Creates 10-12 Crêpes.
Serves 3-12.

Within each category, ingredients flow from easiest to pair to those that invite more thoughtful matching.

Tips on how to apply

Getting Started

All you truly need are ingredients for crêpe batter - everything else is flexible.

- Tools/Equipment: See detailed notes in the previous (Savory Crêpes) framework.

Keeping it Healthy

Focus on fresh fruit, using just a bisou of whipped cream or sauce for a delectable treat that's still light.

Pairings & Balance

This framework is naturally versatile - simply combine complementary flavors and textures you love most.

- Balance Sweet & Tart: Brighten fruits with lemon juice or zest.
- Contrast Textures: Combine creamy spreads with fresh fruit and crunchy nuts or coconut.

Other Tips

- Cooked Fruit: Fresh fruits are delicious - cooking them adds a new dimension of flavor - consider caramelizing bananas, poaching pears, grilling pineapple or sautéing apples with butter and cinnamon.
- Crêpe Cakes: Make mille-crêpes by stacking ~20 crêpes with thin layers of (flavored) whipped cream in between.
- Sweet + Savory: Experiment by mixing sweet and savory, such as bacon & maple syrup, brie & apple, fig jam & prosciutto, or even peach & honey-glazed ham.

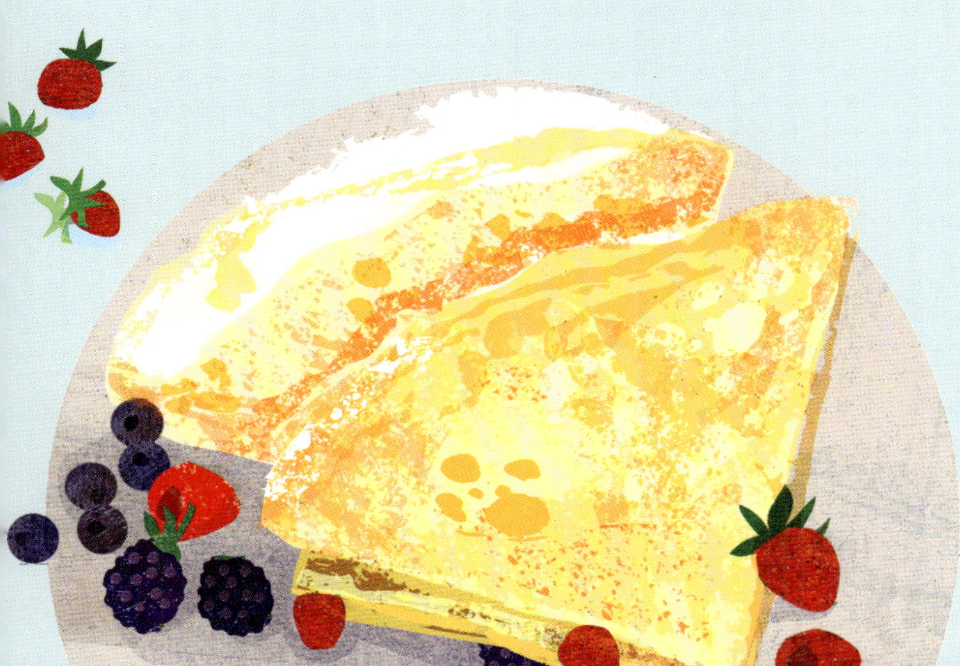

Example pairings

Classic Banana Nutella

Banana, Nutella

Garnish: Hazelnut, Powdered Sugar

Strawberry Cream 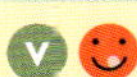

Strawberry, Whipped Cream

Garnish: Mint, Powdered Sugar

Berry Tarragon Medley 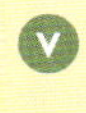

Strawberry, Blackberry and/or Blueberry

Garnish: Honey, Tarragon, Lemon Wedge

Chocolate Orange Delight 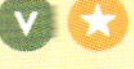

Dried Date, Orange Marmalade, Chocolate Syrup/Nutella; optional: Tangerine slices, Grand Marnier (in batter)

Garnish: Pistachio; optional: Mint

Tropical Coconut Pineapple 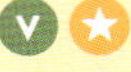

Use Coconut Milk in batter, grilled Pineapple

Garnish: Coconut Flakes, Macadamia, Lime Zest

Peach Ricotta Dream 

Peach, Sweetened Ricotta

Garnish: Basil, Honey

Matcha Mascarpone Strawberry 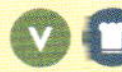

Strawberry, Mascarpone

Garnish: Matcha Powder, Almond

Fundamental Veggies

Sautéed Veggie

Roasted Veggie

Puréed Veggie Soup +Plating Base/Dip

Stuffed Veggie

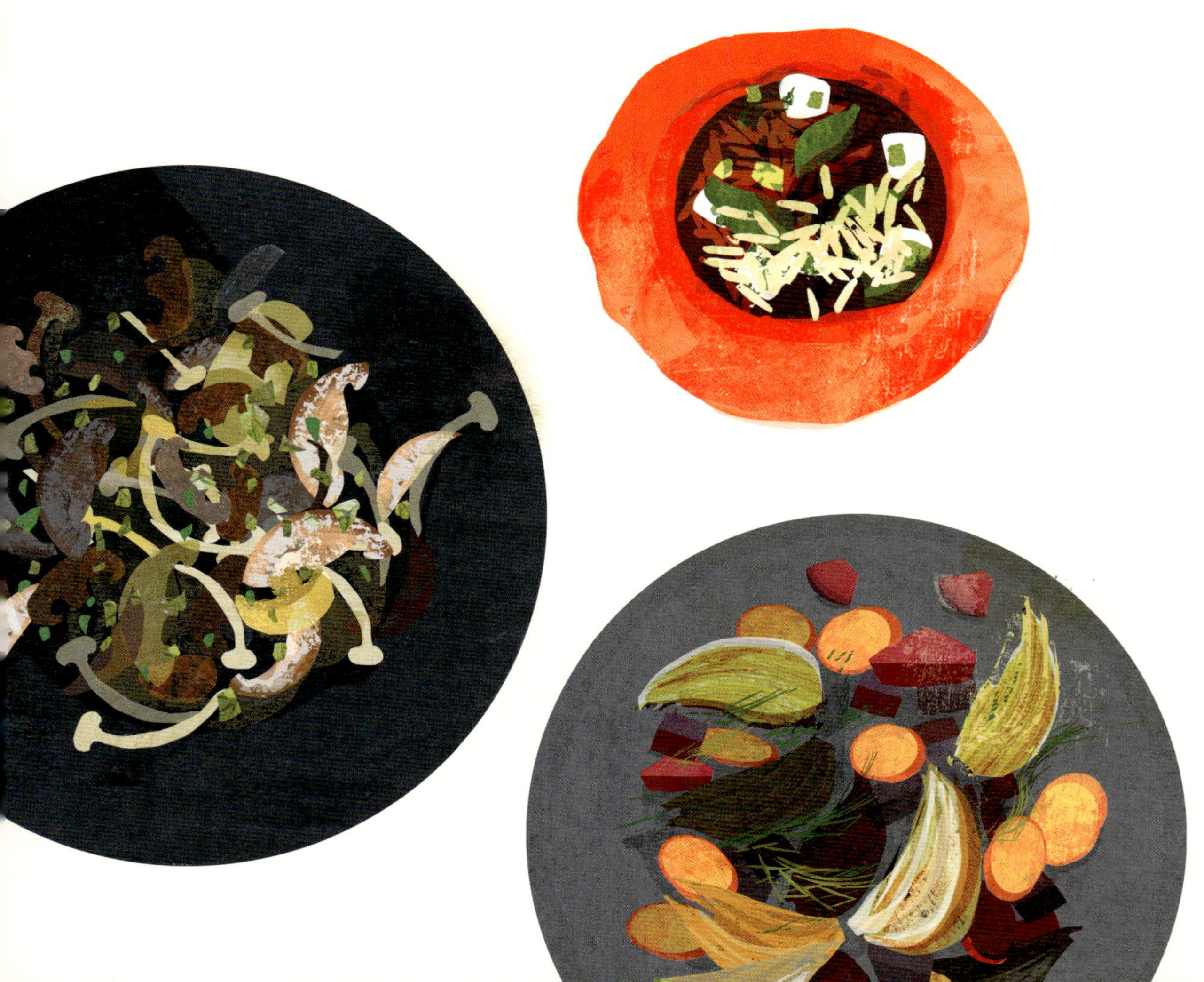

Think of sautéed veggies as a salad with a touch of heat – quick, adaptable, and incredibly customizable. Just like a salad, you can mix and match ingredients, layer flavors, and even chill them for a whole new dimension in grain bowls or cold salads.

Roasting takes things further, deepening flavors and caramelizing natural sugars, while puréeing transforms these elements into silky soups or plating bases.

Master these techniques, and vegetables become more than a side – they become fundamental improvisation.

Sautéed Veggie Framework

Spice up sautéed veggies countless ways or keep it simple - just one vegetable, oil, and seasoning - everything else is optional.

While sautéing may feel like second nature, this framework offers a simple guide for leveling it up. Start with a mix of chopped veggies, then layer in flavor from garlic/ginger, nuts, cheeses, spices, and herbs. Sequence your additions to match cook time, then finish with a splash of acid and a handful of herbs for balance and brightness.

Prep

1. Chop Veggies to a similar size - smaller for faster cooking, larger for easier prep.

- Onion: Brown, White, Red, Shallot - sliced, with the grain
- Aromatic Veggies: Bell Pepper, Fennel, Carrot, Celery, Leek, Parsnip - sliced
- Tomato: Any - chopped & seeded, unless Cherry
- Hearty Veggies: Mushroom, Brussels Sprout, Broccoli, Cauliflower, Eggplant, Zucchini, Cabbage, Kohlrabi - chopped
- Tender Veggies: Green Bean, Snap Peas, Bok Choy, Spinach, Kale, Swiss Chard - whole or chopped

2. Stage other ingredients you're planning to use

Cook

3. Warm large pan on medium or wok on medium-high, with:

- Oil: ~1T Olive Oil, Avocado Oil, Butter, or Bacon (2 oz Bacon = 1T Oil)
- Garlic/Ginger [optional]: Mince and infuse for 30 sec

4. Sauté Veggies, sequencing by category, as earlier categories benefit from longer cook times

5. Boost [optional] with flavor enhancers, in sequence by category:

- Nuts: Pistachio, Cashew, Almond, Pine Nut, Walnut, Peanut, Pecan, Macadamia, Chestnut, Coconut Flakes, Water Chestnut - whole or crushed
- Cheese: Parmesan, Feta, Goat, (smoked) Gouda, Ricotta, Gruyère - grated/crumbled
- Brine: Olive, Caper, Soy Sauce

Finish

6. Season, with Salt & Pepper, plus in sequence by category:

- Spice: Cumin, Coriander, Paprika, Red Pepper Flakes, Cayenne, Turmeric
- Acid: Vinegar (Red Wine, Cider, Balsamic, Rice, Champagne), Citrus Juice/Zest (Lemon, Lime, Orange), Wine

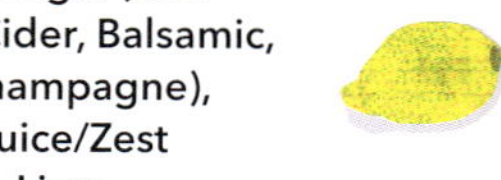

- Herbs: Tarragon, Basil, Oregano, Cilantro, Parsley, Mint, Thyme, Rosemary

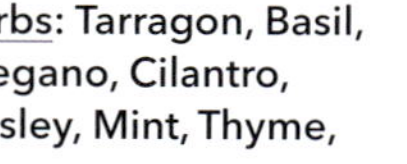

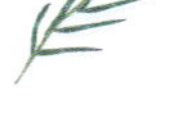

Suggested quantities are per 1 lb of Veggies. Serves 2-6 as a side.

Ingredients flow from easiest to pair to those that benefit from more consideration.

Tips on how to apply

Getting Started

With a well-stocked pantry of herbs, spices, and oils, all you need is to grab whatever veggies look best.

Keeping it Healthy

This is just about as healthy as a dish can be - skip or sparingly use cheese/nuts if looking to keep calories minimal.

Pairings & Balance

You won't go wrong here - either play it safe by sticking to ingredients from a particular region or mix it up to create the latest fusion - some additional suggestions:

- Sweet-Savory: Pair sweeter veggies (carrots, bell peppers, onions) with savory elements (garlic, olives, capers) for contrast.
- Texture: Adding a bit of crunch (from nuts or bacon) is particularly beneficial to mouthfeel when using softer veggies.

Other Tips

- Technique: Let veggies sear to get flavorful browning by limiting stirring and oil use.
- Deglaze Pan: Splash some vinegar, wine, or citrus juice to lift flavors and prevent sticking.
- Uses: Sautéed Veggies work great by themselves as a side dish, can be added to a salad (once closer to room temperature), or transformed into a Soup/Dip/Plating Base (2 frameworks ahead).

Example pairings

Garlic Onion
Olive Oil, Garlic, Yellow Onion

Brussels Sprout with Bacon
Bacon, Brussels Sprout, Balsamic Vinegar

Broccoli Parmesan
Olive Oil, Broccoli and/or Cauliflower, Parmesan, Lemon Juice; optional: Breadcrumbs, Almond

Garlic Mushroom
Olive Oil, Garlic, Cremini or Button Mushroom, Lemon Juice, Parsley

Mediterranean Medley
Olive Oil, Garlic, Red Onion, Bell Pepper, Cherry Tomato, Zucchini, Pine Nut, Feta, Red Pepper Flakes, Lemon Juice, Oregano

Asian Veggie Mix 
Sesame Oil, Garlic, Ginger, Green Onion Whites, Carrot, Shitake, Snow Pea, Bok Choy, Cashew, Soy Sauce, Red Pepper Flakes, Five-Spice, Fennel, Rice Vinegar

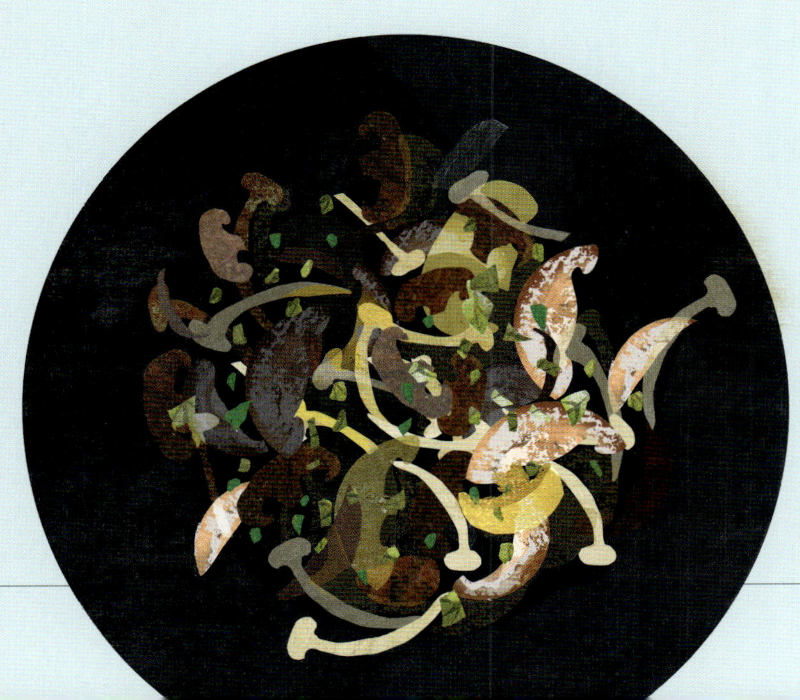

Roasted Veggies Framework

Deepen flavor and crisp texture with this simple, versatile framework.

Roasting draws out rich, caramelized flavors and crisp textures – especially when veggies are cut evenly and seasoned with intention. Start with oil, salt, and pepper, then layer in spices, herbs, or acid for extra dimension. After roasting, finish with cheese, nuts, or fresh herbs to make it shine.

Prep

0. Preheat, oven to 425°F (218 °C)

1. Chop 1-2 lb Veggies of a single type or combo (keep Veggies of different roast times separate)

Long-Roast Veggies (35-45 min)

- Carrots, Parsnip, Turnip, Radish – peeled, whole or sliced
- Cabbage – quartered or cut into eights
- Beet – quartered
- Potato, Sweet Potato, Yam – sliced or whole and pierced
- Butternut Squash, Pumpkin – quartered and seeded

Medium-Roast Veggies (25-35 min)

- Brussels Sprout – halved
- Broccoli, Cauliflower – cut into florets
- Fennel, Leek, Onion (white, yellow) – large slices
- Kohlrabi – peeled, sliced

Quick-Roast Veggies (15-25 min)

- Peppers (any) – quartered and seeded
- Mushroom: Portobello, Cremini, Button, Shiitake, Oyster – whole or quartered
- Eggplant, Zucchini – sliced in 0.5" discs
- Cherry/Grape Tomato - whole, or other Tomatoes – sliced

2. Arrange on lightly oiled baking pan or cookie sheet with some space between

Enhance

Meat [optional]: Wrap around individual Veggies or simply scatter around:

- Prosciutto, Serrano Ham, Bacon

3. Oil: Drizzle over Veggies ~2T:

Olive, Butter, Avocado, Sesame, Neutral or Truffle Oil

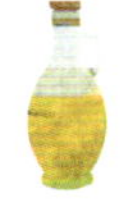

4. Season with Salt & Pepper, and 0-5 additional:

- Garlic: 0-4 cloves – minced
- Spices: 0-1T Coriander, Cumin, Paprika, Sumac, Red Pepper Flakes, Cayenne (lower quantity)

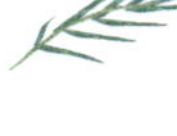

- Dried Herbs: 0-2T Basil, Oregano, Tarragon, Herbes de Provence, Thyme

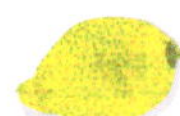

- Acid: 0-2T Vinegar (Balsamic, White Wine) or Citrus Juice (add now or after cooking)

Cook & Finish

5. Roast Veggies according to cook time (listed in step 1)

If combining different types, add quicker-roasting Veggies when the remaining cook time matches their cook time.

6. Garnish, all optional, 0-6T:

- Cheeses: Add in the last few min or right out of the oven to melt: Parmesan, Pecorino Romano, Mozzarella, Cheddar, Goat, Feta – grated/crumbled
- Nuts: Add on top in the last few min of cooking: Pine Nut, Walnut, Almond, Cashew – whole or chopped

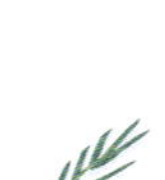

- Herbs: Sprinkle on top just before serving: Basil, Oregano, Parsley, Tarragon, Cilantro, Thyme, Rosemary, Mint – chopped

Serves 2-6 per lb of Veggies, as a side.

Roasted Veggies can also be blended into a smooth, flavorful Soup or Plating Base using the framework that follows.

Tips on how to apply

Getting Started

With a well-stocked pantry of herbs, spices, and oils, all you need is to grab whatever veggies look best.

Keeping it Healthy

This is just about as healthy as a dish can be - sparingly use oil, cheese and nuts if looking to minimize calories.

Pairings & Balance

It's hard to go wrong here - start simple when roasting. You can always zhuzh it up with enhanced garnishes.

- Wrapping with Meat: Cherry tomatoes, okra and asparagus lend themselves particularly well to this.
- Cabbage: Increase the volume of seasonings heavily and consider scattering meat such as prosciutto throughout.

Other Tips

- Convection Oven: Reduce cook time by ~5 min or lower temp 20°F (11°C).
- Broiler: This works more like grilling, so ~15 min may be enough time; works best for veggies that do well grilling, e.g., peppers.
- Chop Sizes: If using multiple different Veggies, cut to relatively similar size for even cooking and cut denser Veggies smaller than less dense Veggies.
- Larger Veggies: Large butternut squash, pumpkin, or whole beets may require increasing cook time to 60 min.
- Uses: Roasted Veggies work great by themselves as a side dish, can be added to a salad, or transformed into a Soup/Dip/Plating Base (see next framework).

Example pairings

Brussels Sprout Bacon

Brussels Sprout, Pancetta/Bacon, Olive Oil, reduced Balsamic Vinegar

Cherry Tomato & Prosciutto

Cherry Tomato, Prosciutto, Olive Oil

Provençal Roasted Root Veggies VV

Any or all of Beet/Carrot/Fennel, Olive Oil, Herbes de Provence, Orange Zest and Juice

Mushroom & Garlic VV

Mushroom, Olive Oil, Garlic

Cauliflower Pine Nut Parmesan V

Cauliflower, Olive Oil, Garlic, Tarragon

Garnish: Lemon Juice, Parmesan and Pine Nuts; optional: Tahini, Chili

Sweet Potato Fig Walnut V

Sweet Potatoes, Olive Oil, Balsamic

Garnish: Fresh Figs, Walnut, Lemon Juice, Feta/Burrata

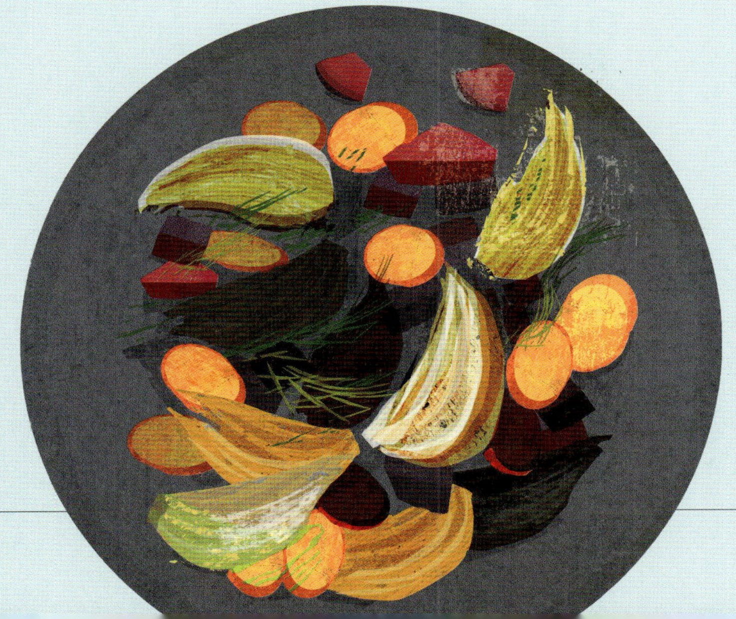

Puréed Veggie Soup Framework with Plating Base Variation

Transform veggies into smooth, expressive forms - from soups to plating art.

This framework builds on your Roasted or Sautéed Veggies - adding just a couple extra steps to turn them into smooth, richly flavored creations. Blend with liquid to your preferred thickness: more for soup, less for a plating base or dip. Serve warm, chilled, or as a vibrant canvas.

Cook

1a. Sauté:

- Follow through Sauté step in Sautéed Veggie Framework (p72)
- Reserve any garnish for the Finish step

OR

1b. Roast:

- Follow through Cook step in Roasted Veggie Framework (p74)
- Set aside any Meat for the Finish step

OR

1c. Boil:

- Chop Veggies (Potato, Yam, Carrot, Parsnip are ideal)
- Simmer 8-14 min in 2c Stock and ~2T Herbs/Spices per lb of Veggies
- Plating Base Variation: Use just enough Stock to cover Veggies

Purée

2. Transfer to blender

3. Add 1-2c Stock per lb of Veggies (if not already added); blend

- Plating Base Variation: Add just enough liquid to puree
- Dairy [optional]: ~0.25c Plain Greek Yogurt, Ricotta, Cream, Sour Cream, Milk, Butter, Coconut Milk or other Dairy substitute

- Acid [optional]: ~0.25c Citrus Juice or Vinegar (avoid combining with Dairy)

4. Season with Salt & Pepper

Finish

5a. Hot Soup:
Heat in pan if needed

OR

5b. Cold Soup:
Refrigerate 2+ hours

OR

5c. Plating Base:
Use as base for Proteins, or serve as a side dish/dip

6. Garnish [optional]

- Any from Sauteed/ Roasted Veggie Frameworks

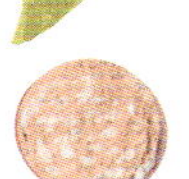

- Soup Favorites: Herbs, Chives, Cheese, Crackers
- Meat: From Roasted Veggies or Meal Prep

Serves 2-6 per lb of Veggies, as a side.

Tips on how to apply

Getting Started

With a well-stocked pantry of herbs, spices, and oils, all you need is to grab some stock and whatever veggies look best.

Keeping it Healthy

Naturally nutrient-dense and packed with fiber, puréed veggie soups are a healthy choice – keep them light by limiting cream and cheese.

- Protein: Add lean meats, lentils or beans for a more complete meal.

Pairings & Balance

- Salt: Stock usually provides considerable salt, so account for that when seasoning; if using water, adjust seasoning accordingly, using more here than for roasted veggies.
- Spices: Generously add pepper and other spices to taste.
- Dairy & Citrus: Use either (or neither – not both) when blending to prevent curdling. Citrus juice creates a lighter, brighter, healthier version – especially refreshing in warm months.

Other Tips

- Cook Time: Larger, denser veggies require longer cook times on the upper end of recommended ranges.
- Cold Soup: Can be prepared a day or two in advance.
- Immersion Blender: If boiling, an immersion blender makes the process easier.
- Grains: Thicken and round out texture by adding cooked rice, quinoa, or other grains when blending.
- Vegetable Stew Variation: Take the Boil path and simply skip puréeing – add a diverse range of veggies in order from firmest to softest so they finish cooking together.

Plating Base Variation

- Adapt this framework into a plating base for proteins, a side dish, or dip by simply using less liquid.

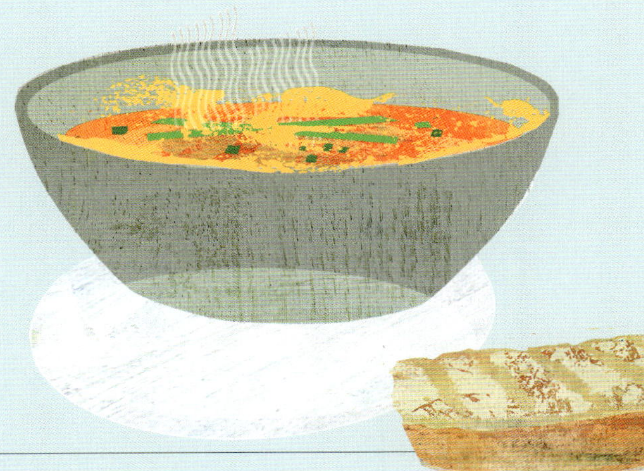

Example pairings

Sautéed Mushroom & Cream Warm Soup

Sauté: Olive Oil, Leek, Garlic, Cremini or mix of Mushrooms, Peppercorn

Blend: Stock, Cream, Tarragon

Roasted Cauliflower Warm Soup

Roast: Cauliflower, Olive Oil, Garlic, Tarragon

Blend: Stock

Garnish: Lemon Juice, Parmesan and Pine Nuts; optional: Chili

(same ingredients as in Roasted Veggies on p74; can start there and create 2 dishes)

Provençal Roasted Root Veggie Cold Soup 

Roast: Any or all of Beet/Carrot/Fennel, Olive Oil, Herbes de Provence, Orange Zest + Juice

Boil: Stock, Cream; Blend

(same ingredients as in Roasted Veggies on p74; can start there and create 2 dishes)

Gazpacho 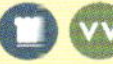

(no cooking or stock needed, just blend)

Tomato, Garlic, Cucumber, Olive Oil, Bread, Lemon Juice, Shallot, White Wine/Sherry/Wine Vinegar; optional: Chili

Boiled Parsnip Plating-base/Dip 

Boil: Parsnip, (Vegetable) Stock

Blend: Olive Oil, Lemon Juice or Cream, Pepper, Sage; optional: Garlic

Roasted Eggplant Plating base/Dip 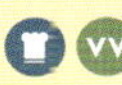

Roast: Eggplant, Garlic, Olive Oil, Salt & Pepper

Blend: Basil, Lemon Juice, Stock

Stuffed Veggie Framework

Craft hearty, delicious vegetable dishes with this broadly adaptable framework.

Stuffed Veggies strike a balance between comfort and creativity – giving you the freedom to repurpose leftovers or invent bold, new combinations. Start by hollowing out a vegetable "vessel," then prepare a flavorful filling and cook it all together. Use contrasting textures and vibrant finishing touches to make each version stand out.

Prep Veggie Vessels

1. Select sturdy Veggie vessels that can be hollowed out or serve as a base, such as:

- Pepper: Bell, Poblano, or Marinated Pimiento*
- Squash: Zucchini, Butternut, Acorn Squash – halved and par-cooked
- Eggplant: Halved and hollowed
- Tomato: Large, firm varieties or Cherry Tomato* – seeded and base cut flat for stability
- Mushroom: Portobello or Cremini – stems removed and sautéed to incorporate in stuffing
- Cabbage: Leaves separated to use as rolls

*Veggies like Marinated Pimiento Pepper and Cherry Tomato can be served cold without cooking

2. Hollow out or halve Veggies, removing seeds/pith/pulp

3. Preheat, oven to 375°F (190°C)

Prep Filling

4. Chop/Pre-Cook as desired:

Grains & Proteins:

- Grains: Quinoa, Rice, Couscous, Farro – cooked; breadcrumbs – toasted
- Proteins: Ground Chicken, Turkey, Beef, Sausage, Tofu – sautéed
- Legumes: Lentil, Chickpea, Black Bean

Core Fillings: Combine with any mix of:

- Veggies: Onion, Tomato, Spinach, Mushroom – diced
- Fruits: Apple, Pear, Peach, Persimmon – diced
- Nuts & Seeds: Pine Nut, Sunflower Seed, Walnut, Almond, Cashew, Pecan - chopped
- Cheeses: Feta, Goat, Parmesan, Mozzarella

- Egg: Whisked (helps with binding)

5. Season with Salt & Pepper, plus any:

- Herbs: 0-4T Parsley, Basil, Oregano, Thyme, Mint, Rosemary, Sage
- Spices: 0-2T Cumin, Paprika, Coriander, Garlic, Onion Powder, Five-Spice, Cardamom, Nutmeg, Cayenne, Turmeric
- Oil: 0-1T Olive, Sesame, Butter

If using ground Proteins, add Spices while sautéing

Stuff-Cook-Finish

6. Fill Veggie Vessels generously, without overpacking

7. Bake at 375°F (190°C) for 20-30 min, until filling is heated through and Veggies are tender

8. Garnish [optional] and return to oven briefly for browning/melting:

- Nuts - crushed
- Cheeses - grated
- Sauces: Marinara, Tahini, Yogurt Sauce, Aioli, Sour Cream

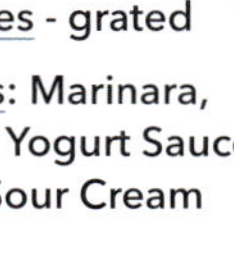

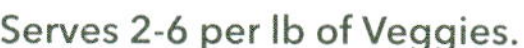

Serves 2-6 per lb of Veggies.

Tips on how to apply

Getting Started

As long as you have "vessel vegetables," you can make this with whatever you have on hand – including repurposed leftovers. This dish is as flexible as it is delicious.

Keeping it Healthy

Naturally nutrient-rich – to maximize healthiness:

- Filling: Include veggies (spinach, mushrooms, or zucchini), to lighten the dish while boosting nutrients.
- Cheese: Use sparingly for flavor.
- Protein: Opt for lean options like chicken, turkey, or plant-based proteins (e.g., lentils).
- Whole Grains: Swap refined grains for quinoa or brown rice to add fiber and nutrients.

Pairings & Balance

Change the flavor profile with global seasonings, e.g.,

- Italian: Oregano, Basil, Thyme, Rosemary
- Greek: Oregano, Garlic Powder, Onion Powder
- Middle Eastern (Ras-el-hanout): Coriander, Cumin, Turmeric, Cinnamon, Allspice
- Mexican (Adobo): Paprika, Garlic, Oregano, Cumin); or Tajín: Chili, Lime, Salt
- Indian (Garam Masala): Cinnamon, Cloves, Cardamom, Cumin
- Chinese (Five-Spice): Star Anise, Cloves, Cinnamon, Fennel, Pepper (+Ginger)
- French (Herbes de Provence): Thyme, Rosemary, Lavender, Savory, Marjoram

Other Tips

- Make Ahead: Prep and stuff veggies in advance – bake just before serving for easy meal prep.

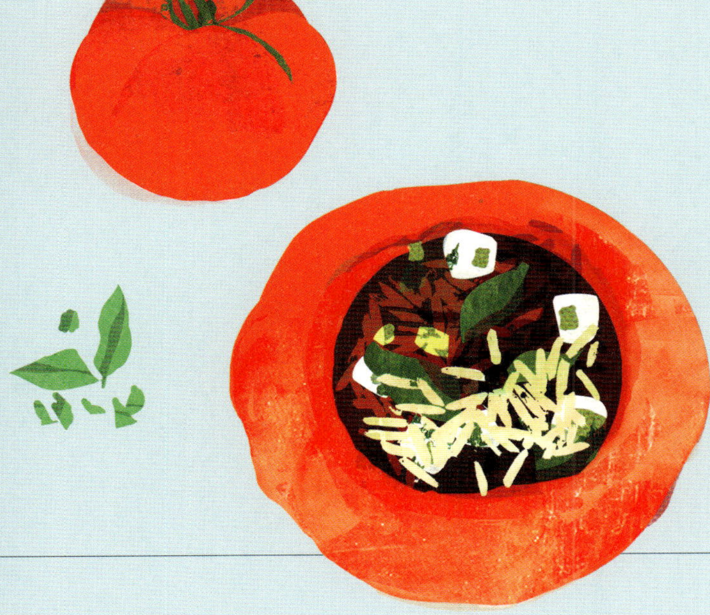

Example pairings

Butternut Squash Apple Walnut

Pre-Roast: Butternut Squash, ~25 min

Stuff Squash with: Faro, Onion, Apple, Walnut, Sage, Nutmeg; **Bake**

Garnish: Yogurt Sauce

Stuffed Mushrooms

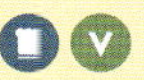

Prep: Cremini Mushrooms, keep Caps whole, remove and chop Stems

Sauté: Garlic, Chopped Stems, Slivered Almonds, Breadcrumbs, Onion Powder, Paprika, Salt & Pepper

Stuff Caps with: Above mixture, topped with Parmesan; **Bake**

Poblano Chili

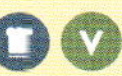

Broil: Poblano Chili, ~15 min; steam-peel

Stuff Chili with: Rice, Black Beans, Onion, Tomato, Zucchini, Garlic, Cayenne, Cilantro; **Bake**

Garnish: Parmesan; optional: Sour Cream

Inverse Bruschetta Caprese

Sauté: Garlic, Onion, Mushroom

Stuff Roma Tomato with: Sautéed Veggies, Breadcrumbs, Prosciutto, Basil, Red Pepper Flakes, Mozzarella; **Broil**

Garnish: Balsamic Glaze, Basil

Korean Stuffed Peppers (Gochu Jeon)

Prep: Bell or Gochu Pepper

Sauté: Ground Pork, Sesame Oil, Ginger, Garlic

Stuff Bell or Gochu Pepper with: Rice, Green Onion, Kimchi, Soy Sauce

Steam or dip in Egg and pan-fry

Pimiento Peppers (cold)

Whole (jarred) marinated Pimiento Pepper

Stuff Peppers with: Garlic, Lemon, Goat or Cottage Cheese, Black Olive, Salt & Pepper; optional: Parsley

Foundational Proteins

Meal Prep

Foundational Chicken

Foundational Beef

Foundational Salmon

Foundational Shrimp

Foundational Pork

Foundational Tofu

Marinated-Roast Chicken

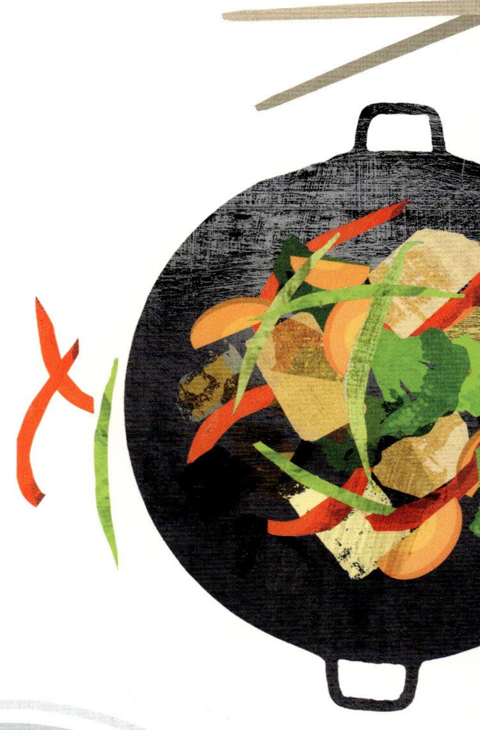

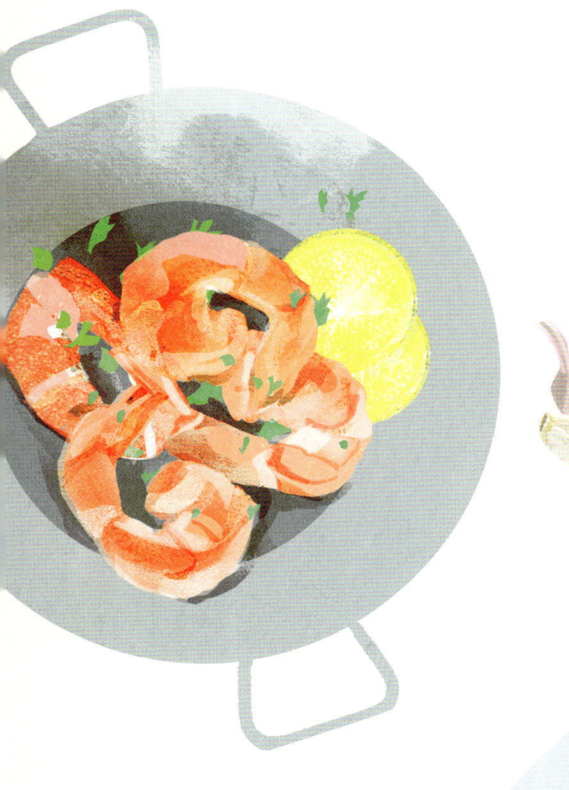

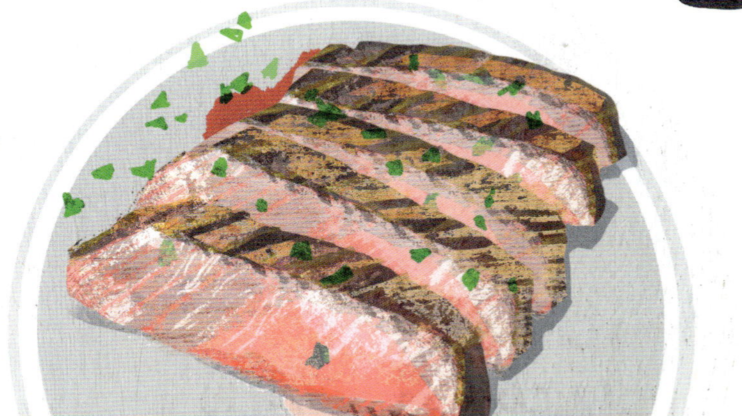

Most CookImprov frameworks start with a method and explore ingredient variations. Here, we flip the script – start with a key ingredient (meat, seafood, or tofu) and explore multiple methods.

These Foundational frameworks are ideal for Meal Prep or quick, go-to weeknight meals. Cook in batches, mix and match seasonings, and pair with a simple salad for a nutrient-packed, effortless foundation that adapts to any meal.

Equipped with these techniques, you'll have freedom to cook based on what's available – choosing whatever inspires you, knowing you can bring any proteins and veggies together with finesse.

Meal Prep

The practice of cooking proteins in advance to set up for quick, healthy meals throughout the week. It's efficient, drives lean protein intake, and opens a wide range of dishes to keep everything feeling fresh:

	Breakfast → Lunch
Classic	Scrambled Egg, Bagel Sandwich, Omelet
Global Fusion	Avocado Toast, Lettuce Wrap
Latin	Bkfst. Burrito, Quesadilla
Asia-Pacific	Spring Roll
Italian	Frittata

Dinner

Sandwich
Soup
Salad
Stuffed Veggies
Flatbread Wrap
Crêpe
Grain Bowl
Nachos
Taco
Burrito
Quinoa Salad
Hawaiian Bowl
Fried Rice
Stir-Fry*
Soba Salad
Pasta Salad
Pizza*
Pasta*
Risotto*

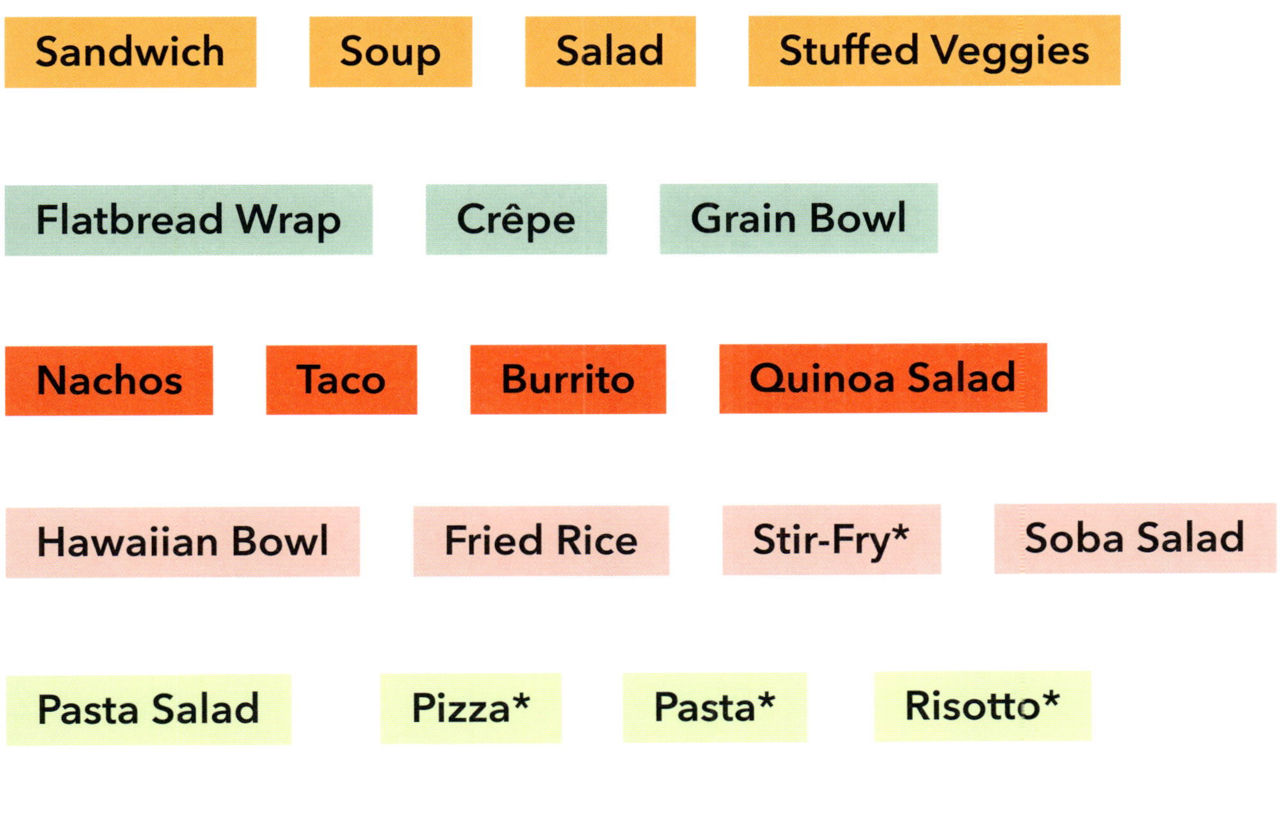

*While Meal Prep proteins can be added to these dishes, the time savings is greatest for dishes that otherwise require little/no cooking

The "Foundational" frameworks that follow are all well-suited for Meal Prep or can be complete meals in and of themselves.

Foundational Chicken Framework

Build flavor and variety into your week with this endlessly adaptable chicken framework.

Start with your preferred form: bite-sized pieces, ground, or flattened cutlets, then choose a stovetop sauté or quick grill. Layer in herbs, spices, or aromatics, and finish with citrus or fresh herbs to brighten. This foundational framework makes it easy to cook once and remix across salads, bowls, wraps, and more throughout the week.

Prep

1. Chicken: Select 2 lb boneless-skinless Breast, Tenders, or Thighs - prepare as:

- Bite-Sized: Chopped evenly
- Flattened: Pounded with meat tenderizer
- Ground

2. Season with Salt & Pepper, plus [optional] ~4T any combo you desire of:

- Aromatics
- Herbs
- Spices

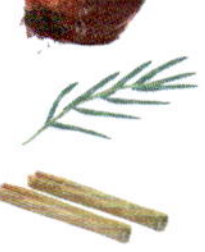

Cook

3a. Pan: Heat 1-2T Oil in pan on medium, then:

- Bite-Sized: Sauté until no pink remains when splitting largest piece ~9 min
- Flattened: Cook 3 min on 1st side, 3 min on 2nd, then ~5 min on 1st side until internal temp reaches 165°F (74°C)
- Ground: Sauté until no pink remains ~7 min
  [optional] Caramelize Onion before adding Chicken; simmer other Veggies along with Chicken

OR

3b. Grill: Brush grill with Oil on high heat:

- Flattened**:** Cook ~4 min per side, until internal temp reaches 165°F (74°C)

Finish

4. Garnish as desired with:

- Fresh Herbs
- Citrus Juice: Lemon, Lime, Orange

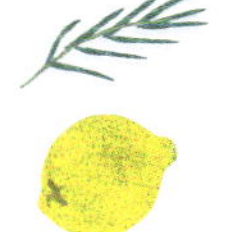

Add just before serving or refrigerate Chicken to add to other dishes throughout the week

Suggested Ingredients

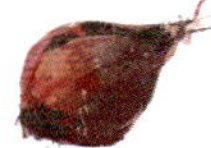

Aromatics

Garlic, Ginger, Shallot, Onion, Chili Pepper - diced

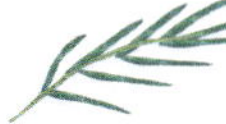

Herbs

Basil,Tarragon, Oregano, Thyme, Rosemary, Mint, Herbes de Provence, Italian Seasoning

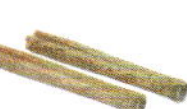

Spices

Paprika, Garlic/Onion Powder, Cumin, Coriander, Mustard, Ras-el-Hanout, Cajun Spices, Jerk Seasoning, Tandoori Blend, Chili Powder

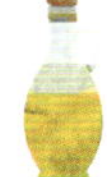

Oil

Olive, Sesame, Avocado*, Canola*, Grapeseed*

**High smoke point oils ideal for grilling*

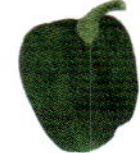

Veggies

Yellow Onion, Shallot, Carrot, Cremini, Shiitake, Button Mushroom, Tomato, Bell Pepper - sliced

Tips on how to apply

Getting Started

All you need is chicken - everything else is flexible or a pantry staple.

Keeping it Healthy

This dish is naturally healthy - just moderate the oil and aim to pair with leafy greens or other veggies for a balanced, nutrient-dense meal.

Pairings & Balance

Simple works well - use herbs, spices, and oils from the same region to keep flavors harmonious.

- Seasoning: Ground chicken typically benefits from more generous seasoning than other cuts - salt, pepper, and spice help it shine.

Meal Prep Ideas

Chicken works especially well in: Salads, Avocado Toast, Crêpes, Soups, Grain Bowls, Flatbread Wraps - even Stuffed Veggies (with ground chicken).

Other Tips

- Tenderizing: Flattening chicken breasts with a meat tenderizer helps reduce cooking time and encourages even doneness.
- Thick Cuts: For especially thick chicken breasts, consider butterflying or slicing in half before cooking to avoid dry exteriors and undercooked centers.
- Meal Prep Basic: The simplest combo (Chicken Breast, Salt, Pepper, Olive Oil), makes a flexible foundation to support other dishes - layer in additional seasonings as desired for specific meals.
- Reheating: Ground chicken or bite-sized pieces reheat most easily; for meals within a few days, chilled chicken also works well in salads or sandwiches.
- Grilling: Grilling adds smokiness and caramelization that elevates flavor without added fat - it's especially effective for marinated cuts, whether whole breasts, thighs, or skewered pieces.

Example pairings

Meal Prep Basic

Chicken Breast, Salt & Pepper, Olive Oil; Lemon (optional)

Garlic Lemon

Chicken Breast, Salt & Pepper, Garlic, Olive Oil, Lemon

Mediterranean

Chicken Breast, Salt & Pepper, Ras-el-Hanout, Garlic, Onion [optional], Olive Oil, Lemon

Latin

Chicken Thighs, Salt & Pepper, Chili, Avocado Oil, Lime

Garlic Ginger

Ground Chicken, Salt & Pepper, Garlic, Ginger, Sesame Oil

Dijon 

Chicken Breast, Salt & Pepper, Garlic, Shallot, Tarragon, Mustard, Olive Oil, Lemon

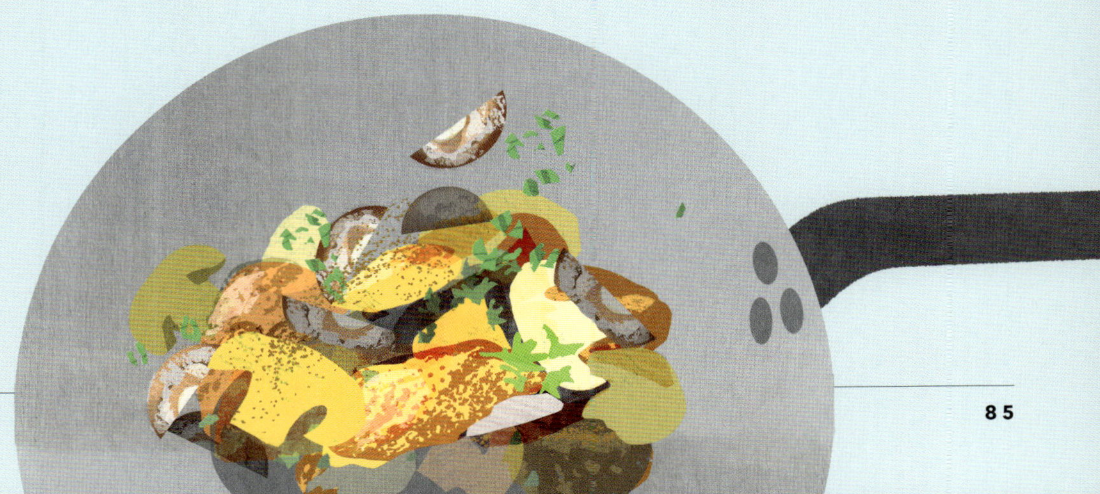

Foundational Beef Framework

Unleash beef's flavor potential with a framework that flexes across cuts, cuisines, and cooking styles.

Start by selecting a cut – thinly sliced, ground, or whole steak – then choose your method: sauté or grill. Use seasonings and umami boosts to layer depth, then finish with herbs or acid to brighten. This flexible framework makes it easy to cook once and enjoy bold, varied meals throughout the week.

Prep

1. Beef: Select 2 lb:

- Thinly Sliced: Beef Flank, Sirloin, Skirt, Round or Chuck
- Ground
- Steaks: Strip, Filet Mignon, Rib Eye, T-Bone

2. Season with Salt & Pepper, plus [optional] ~3T any combo you desire of:

- Aromatics
- Herbs
- Spices
- Umami Boosts

Cook

3a. Pan: Heat 1-2T Oil in pan on medium, then:

- Thinly Sliced: Sauté until browned ~3 min
- Ground: Sauté until no pink remains ~5 min
  [optional] Caramelize Onion and/or Pepper before adding Beef; simmer other Veggies along with Beef
- Steaks: Cook 3 min on 1st side, 3 min on 2nd side, then ~3 min on 1st side until internal temp reaches 130°F (54°C) for medium rare to 145°F (63°C) [USDA recommended]

OR

3b. Grill: Brush grill with Oil on high heat:

- Steaks: Cook ~4 min per side, until internal temp reaches 130°F (54°C) for medium rare to 145°F (63°C) [USDA recommended]

Finish

4. Garnish as desired with:

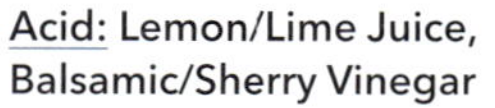

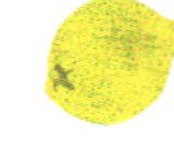

- Acid: Lemon/Lime Juice, Balsamic/Sherry Vinegar
- Fresh Herbs: Parsley, Cilantro, Basil, Chives – chopped
- Crisp: Toasted Sesame Seed, Fried Shallot, or Toasted Crushed Nuts

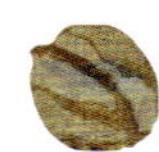

Add just before serving or refrigerate Beef to add to other dishes throughout the week

Suggested Ingredients

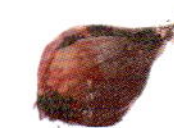

Aromatics

Garlic, Shallot, Onion, Chili Pepper, Ginger – diced

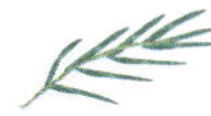

Herbs

Basil, Tarragon, Oregano, Thyme, Rosemary, Mint, Herbes de Provence, Italian Seasoning

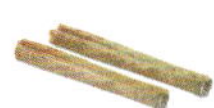

Spices

Paprika, Garlic/ Onion Powder, Cumin, Coriander, Mustard, Ras-el-Hanout, Cajun Spices, Jerk Seasoning, Tandoori Blend, Chili Powder

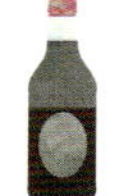

Umami Boosts

Worcestershire Sauce, Soy Sauce, Fish Sauce, Miso Paste

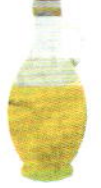

Oil

Olive, Sesame, Avocado*, Canola*, Grapeseed*

*High smoke point oils ideal for grilling

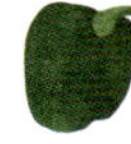

Veggies

Yellow Onion, Shallot, Carrot, Cremini, Shiitake, Button Mushroom, Tomato, Bell Pepper – sliced

Yields ~4 meals.

Tips on how to apply

Getting Started

All you need is beef - everything else is flexible or a pantry staple.

Keeping it Healthy

Opt for sirloin, round, or trimmed chuck - they deliver great flavor with less fat.

- Ground Beef: 90%+ lean is healthiest and tastes great if well-seasoned; 85% lean offers a good balance.
- Oil: Favor olive/avocado oil over butter to keep things lighter while delivering richness - either way, less is needed when using beef with higher fat content.

Pairings & Balance

It's fine to keep things simple - using herbs, spices, and oils from the same region or cuisine generally ensures a harmonious flavor profile.

- Seasoning: Ground beef typically benefits from more generous seasoning than other cuts - extra salt, pepper, and spices help bring out its full flavor.

Meal Prep Ideas

Beef works especially well in: Sandwiches, Grain Bowls, Hawaiian Protein Bowls, Salads, Soups, Tacos - even Stuffed Veggies (with ground beef).

Other Tips

- Meal Prep Basic: The simplest combo (bite-sized beef, salt, pepper, garlic powder, olive oil), makes a flexible foundation to support other dishes - layer in additional seasonings as desired for specific meals.
- Cutting: Slice against the grain for tenderness - especially important for thin strips.
- Reheating: Ground or cubed beef reheats easily - chilled leftovers also work well in wraps, salads, or sandwiches.
- Baking Soda: Add 0.25-0.5t (dissolved in water) per lb of meat to boost browning - especially for ground meat; it's not a panacea, as it converts acids to salt - so adjust seasoning and add citrus/vinegar at the end to balance.

Example pairings

Meal Prep Basic

Salt, Pepper, Garlic Powder, Olive Oil

Classic Italian Herb

Garlic, Italian Seasoning, Onion Powder, Olive Oil, Shallot

Garnish: Basil, Balsamic Vinegar, Parmesan

Smoky Southwestern

Smoked Paprika, Cumin, Garlic Powder, Worcestershire Sauce, Chili Flakes, Olive Oil, Shallot

Garnish: Parsley, Lime

Caribbean Jerk Style

Garlic, Jerk Seasoning, Paprika, Cayenne, Avocado Oil, Shallot

Garnish: Cilantro, Lime

Thai Chili

Garlic, Ginger, Peanut/Neutral Oil, Shallot, Chili Pepper; optional: Fish Sauce

Garnish: Thai Basil, Peanut

Korean Sesame Soy

Garlic, Ginger, Red Pepper Flakes, Soy Sauce, Toasted Sesame Oil, Green Onion

Garnish: Sesame Seed, Sherry Vinegar

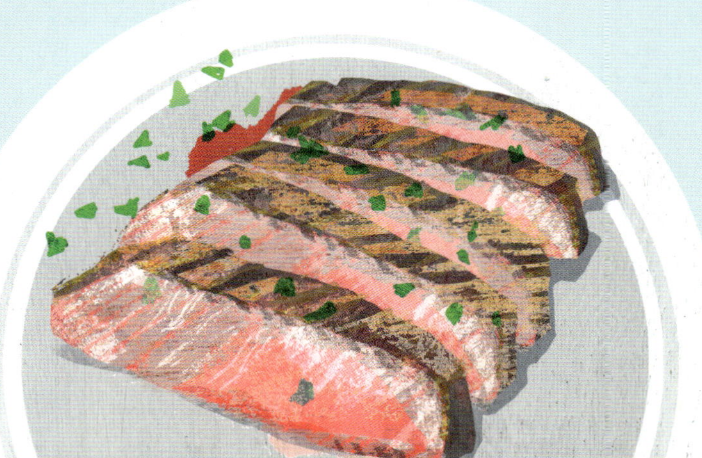

Foundational Pork Framework

Unlock pork's rich versatility with this simple, adaptable framework - ideal for meal prep and weeknights, whether on the stovetop or grill.

Start with your preferred cut, then choose between a quick sauté or skewered grill. Use the optional sauce to build flavor through marinating or finishing. With a broad palette of spices, herbs, acids, and sweeteners, this flexible framework supports bold, balanced combinations that carry across multiple meals.

Prep

1. Pork: Select 2 lb boneless:

- Thinly Sliced: Shoulder, Loin, Tenderloin - cut against the grain
- Ground

2. Season with Salt & Pepper, plus any desired Seasonings

Sauce [optional: for marinade or finishing]

Whisk together:

- Oil: 2-3T Olive, Sesame or Neutral
- Acid: 2-3T
- Seasonings: ~2T - ground
- Salt & Pepper
- Sweet [optional]: 1-2T

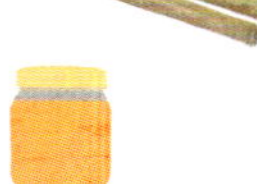

Cook

3a. Pan/Wok, on high heat:

- Heat 2-4T Oil: Neutral, Olive Oil, or Butter
  Veggies/Fruits [optional]: Chop and briefly sauté
- Add Pork, sauté ~4 min, stirring occasionally - should be browned, no pink remaining
  Wine [optional]: Deglaze with ~2T, Sherry, Port, Bourbon, or Calvados

OR

3b. Grill Satay-style, skewered, on high heat

- Soak wooden skewers in water to prevent burning; skewer Pork
- Heat grill, brush with high smoke point Neutral Oil
- Add Pork, grill ~4 min, brush with marinade or Oil; flip and grill another ~2 min

Finish

4. Garnish as desired with:

- Herbs
- Acid
- Sauce
- Nuts: crushed, roasted

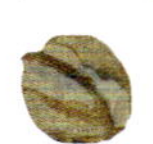

Add just before serving or refrigerate Pork to add to other dishes throughout the week

Suggested Ingredients

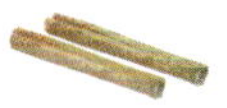

Seasonings

Garlic, Ginger, Paprika, Cumin, Coriander, Dijon, Soy Sauce, Chili, Fennel, Star Anise, Clove, Cinnamon, Hoisin, Turmeric

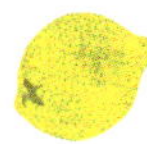

Acid

Citrus Juice (Orange, Lemon, Lime) or Vinegar (Balsamic, Red Wine, Cider, Sherry, White Wine, Rice)

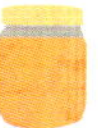

Sweet

Sugar, Maple Syrup, Honey, Fruit Preserves, Juice (Orange, Apple, Pineapple)

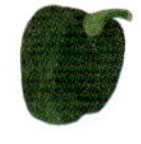

Veggies

Onion (Green, Sweet, Red, Yellow, White), Shallot, Bell Pepper, Tomato, Carrot, Cabbage, Shiitake, Cremini, Sweet Potato, Potato, Pea, Snow Pea, Turnip

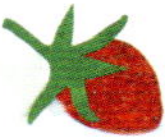

Fruits

Pineapple, Apple, Mango, Peach, Apricot, Pear, Persimmon

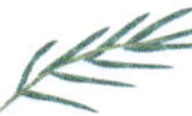

Herbs

Parsley, Cilantro, Rosemary, Oregano, Thyme, Green Onion Greens, Mint, Sage, Basil, Marjoram

Yields ~4 meals.

Tips on how to apply

Getting Started

All you need is pork - everything else is flexible or a pantry staple.

Keeping it Healthy

While Pork has a reputation for being unhealthy, fat content varies widely by cut - opt for lean cuts such as loin or tenderloin - they're leaner than most cuts of beef and even comparable to chicken.

Pairings & Balance

It's fine to keep things simple - using herbs, spices and oils from one culinary region (Latin, Asian, Mediterranean) creates reliably harmonious flavors.

Meal Prep Ideas

Pork works especially well in: Salads, Hawaiian Protein Bowls, Lettuce Wraps, Spring Rolls, Tacos, Scrambled Eggs.

Other Tips

- Quick Marinade: Pork loin and tenderloin benefit from even short marinades (20-30 minutes), due to their mild flavor and leaner profile.
- Avoid Overcooking: Pork dries out quickly - cook just until no pink remains, internal temp of 145°F (63°C).
- Rest: Briefly rest pork after cooking to retain juices.
- Meal Prep Basic: The simplest combo (pork, salt, pepper, olive oil), makes a flexible foundation to support other dishes - layer in additional seasonings or sauces for specific meals.
- Reheating: Ground or bite-sized pork reheats most easily.

Example pairings

Meal Prep Basic

Salt, Pepper, Olive Oil; optional: Orange

Dijon Apple

Dijon Mustard, Garlic, Thyme, Apple Cider Vinegar

Pan: Sweet Onion, Apple, Cremini

Garnish: Parsley

Maple Bourbon

Smoked Paprika, Garlic, Thyme, Apple Cider Vinegar, Maple Syrup

Pan: Shallot, Sweet Potato (parboiled), Bourbon

Garnish: Parsley, Pecan

Chili Lime

Garlic, Cumin, Coriander, Chili Powder/Cayenne

Pan: Red Onion, Bell Pepper

Garnish: Cilantro, Lime, optional: sliced Avocado

Satay with Peanut Sauce

Marinate: Coconut Cream, Lime Juice, Ginger, Sugar, Coriander, Cumin, Turmeric

Grill: Neutral Oil with high smoke point

Dipping Sauce: Peanut Butter, Lime Juice, Soy Sauce, Garlic, Ginger, Sugar, water to dilute; optional: Chili Paste

Orange Clove

Garlic, Clove, Cinnamon, Coriander

Pan: Sweet Onion, Apple, Cremini

Garnish: Orange Zest, Parsley or Cilantro

Soy Ginger Honey

Ginger, Garlic, Soy Sauce, Honey, Rice Vinegar

Pan: Green Onion Whites, Shiitake

Garnish: Green Onion Greens

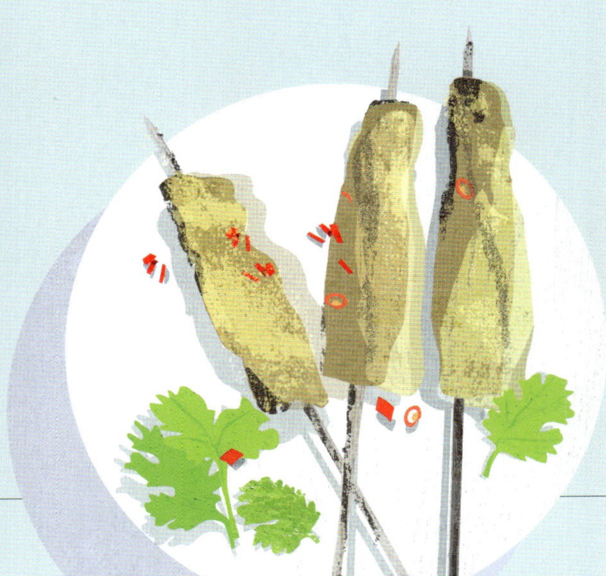

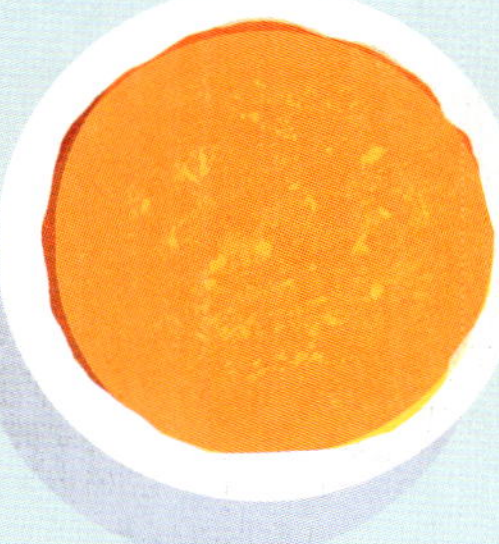

Foundational Fish Framework

Fuel your week with this fish dish that's lean, fast, and flavorful.

Start with a firm, richly textured fish such as salmon, then choose between a quick pan-fry or a simple grilled preparation. Explore the wide range of spices, herbs, veggies, and acid to craft colorful combinations. Use the optional sauce as a marinade or finishing drizzle. Enjoy warm, and/or refrigerate to mix into grain bowls, salads, wraps, or other meals throughout the week.

Prep

1. Fish: Select 2 lb fillet of Salmon or similar

- For Pan: Remove skin and bones, cut into 0.5-1″ cubes
- For Grill: Rinse and pat dry

2. Season with Salt & Pepper, plus any desired Spices

Sauce [optional]:
Whip together a sauce that can either be used as a marinade or added to fish at the end:

- Oil: 2-6T Olive, Avocado, Sesame or Neutral
- Acid: 2-3T Citrus Juice or Vinegar
- Garlic - minced
- Spices: ~2T - ground
- Salt & Pepper

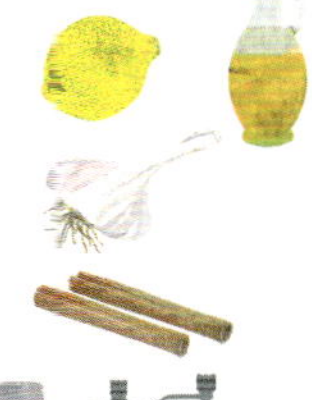

Cook

3a. Pan, on medium heat:

- Heat 1-2T Oil: Olive, Butter, Neutral
  Veggies [optional]: Chop and sauté; remove if needed
- Sauté Fish 4-6 min, stirring occasionally
  Wine [optional]: Deglaze with ~2T Wine, Sherry, or Sake

OR

3b. Grill, on medium-high:

- Grill 5 min skin-side down
- Flip and grill another ~1 min - 120°F (49°C) for Medium Rare, 145°F (63°C) for USDA recommended doneness

Finish

4. Check doneness:

- Will flake when pierced with a fork, if fully cooked

5. Garnish as desired with:

- Herbs
- Acid
- Sauce
- Nuts: crushed, roasted

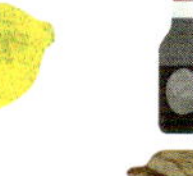

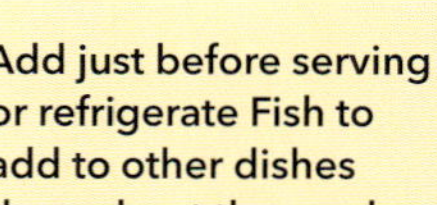

Add just before serving or refrigerate Fish to add to other dishes throughout the week

Suggested Ingredients

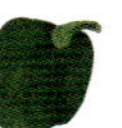

Veggies

Shallot, Onion (Red, White), Tomato, Cremini, Carrot, Fennel, Leek, Olive, Caper, Potato, Daikon, Celery, Kale

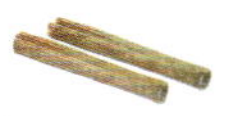

Spices

Red Pepper Flakes, Paprika, Ginger, Fennel, Coriander, Cumin, Saffron, Lemongrass, Turmeric, Cardamom, Teriyaki

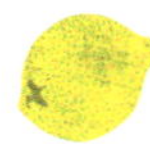

Acid

Citrus Juice (Lemon, Lime, Orange, Grapefruit, Yuzu) or Vinegar (White Wine, Balsamic, Sherry, Rice, Cider)

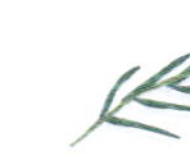

Herbs

Parsley, Tarragon, Basil, Mint, Dill, Thyme, Green Onion Greens, Chives, Cilantro, Shiso, Marjoram

Yields ~4 meals.

Tips on how to apply

Getting Started

All you need is fish – everything else is flexible or a pantry staple.

Keeping it Healthy

This dish is naturally healthy thanks to the lean protein and omega-3s in fish – just be mindful of any oil or sugar in the glaze/sauce.

Pairings & Balance

Each fish has its own affinities – use these quick pairings as inspiration when building out flavor beyond Salmon:

- Artic Char, Steelhead Trout: Closest to Salmon; flavor affinities largely overlap
- Mahi Mahi*: Lemon, Orange, Coriander, Cilantro, White Pepper, Tomato, Mango
- Sea Bass: Lime, Lemon, Shiitake, Coriander, Cilantro, Shiso, Shallot, Daikon
- Cod: Lemon, Basil, Chives, Miso, Togarashi, Saffron, Cayenne, Carrot, Tomato
- Halibut*: Lemon, Lime, Garlic, Ginger, Cilantro, Fennel, Coriander, Chives, Leek

Meal Prep Ideas

Fish works especially well in: Hawaiian Protein Bowls, Salads, Soups, Quinoa Bowls, Lettuce Wraps.

Other Tips

- Meal Prep Basic: The simplest combo (fish, olive oil, garlic, citrus zest and juice) makes a flexible foundation to support other dishes – layer in additional seasonings as desired for specific meals.
- Grilling: For best results, baste with oil or marinade while grilling to add flavor and prevent sticking; keep skin-on for easier handling on the grill.
    - Salmon particularly benefits from the smokiness of grilling.
- Roasting: Heat oven to 450°F (232°C), cook for 5 min on one side, flip and cook ~4 on the other, otherwise following the same approach as Grilling.
- Salmon Skin: If you've removed the skin to pan-fry the fish, crisp it in a dry pan over medium heat, flipping occasionally; once crisp, chop it up – it's like a healthier version of bacon bits and pairs beautifully with lightly dressed arugula.
- Reheating: Fish is excellent chilled in grain bowls or salads; if reheating, do so gently: covered, on low heat or in the microwave to avoid drying out.

*Unlike Salmon, avoid eating the skin of these fish.

Example pairings

Meal Prep Basic

Pan-Fry: Salmon, Olive Oil, Garlic, Lime Zest + Juice

Tapa Style

Pan: Salmon, Olive Oil

Sauce: Olive Oil, Sherry Vinegar, Paprika, Cumin

Garnish: Parsley

Lemon Balsamic

Salmon, Garlic, Oregano

Pan: Olive Oil, Shallot, Cherry Tomato,

Garnish: Basil, Lemon Zest + Juice, Reduced Balsamic

Caribbean Lime Spice

Mahi Mahi, Allspice, Red Pepper Flakes

Pan: Neutral Oil, Garlic, Red Onion

Garnish: Cilantro, Lime Wedge

Salmon Teriyaki

Marinate: Salmon, Garlic, Ginger, Teriyaki Sauce, Rice Vinegar, Mirin

Grill

Garnish: Green Onion Greens, Sesame Seed

CI take on: Nobu Style Miso Black Cod

Marinate: Black Cod, White Miso, Mirin, Sake, Sugar, Ginger (warm marinade to dissolve Miso) – marinate 1-3 days, then brush off

Pan-Sear: Neutral Oil

Garnish: Sesame Oil, Green Onion Greens, Lemon Wedge

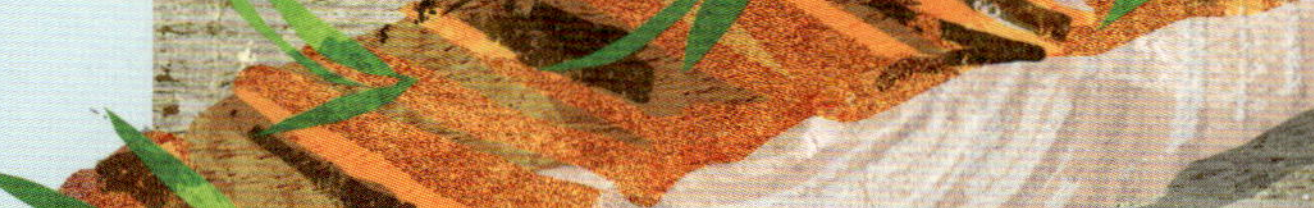

Foundational Shrimp Framework

With key components so simple, you're likely to learn by heart – revisit when craving new variations.

Choose a low-oil sauté, a high-oil infusion for dipping, or grill for a smoky finish. From quick weeknight meals to bold, elegant plates, small variations yield strikingly different results.

Prep

1. Shrimp: Select 2 lb, medium to jumbo

- Remove legs and devein
- Remove shells for easier eating, or leave on to retain moisture (especially when grilling) – tails can stay either way

Cook

2a. Pan, on medium heat:

- Heat 2-12T Oil: Olive, Butter, Neutral
- Add minced Garlic and 0-2T Spices
  Veggies [optional]: Chop and sauté 1 min
- Add Shrimp, sauté 2-5 min (medium-jumbo), flip halfway
  Wine [optional]: Deglaze with ~2T Wine, Sherry, Sake, or Pastis

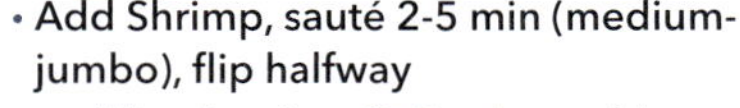

The high vs. low oil decision branches into two distinct styles of dish: in the low-oil version, the oil simply cooks the shrimp; in the high-oil version, the shrimp infuses the oil with rich flavor, perfect for dipping bread

OR

2b. Grill, on medium-high, skewered:

- Toss Shrimp with Oil, Garlic, and Spices
- Skewer and grill 1-2 min per side

Finish

3. Check doneness:

- Shrimp are done when opaque and firm, curled into a loose "C" shape
- Avoid overcooking: (tight "O" shape = rubbery texture)

4. Season and garnish:

- Citrus Juice + Zest
- Herbs

Suggested Ingredients

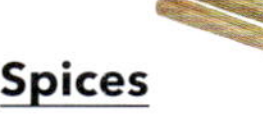

Spices

Red Pepper Flakes, Paprika, Fennel Seed, Saffron, Ginger, Five-Spice, Coriander, Cumin, Lemongrass, Star Anise

Veggies

Onion, Shallot, Fennel, Tomato, Bell Pepper, Carrot, Celery, Leek, Shiitake, Chanterelle

Citrus

Lemon, Lime, Orange, Yuzu

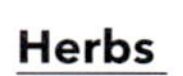

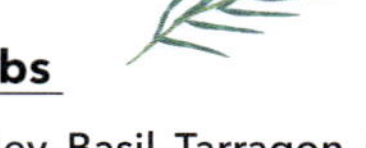

Herbs

Parsley, Basil, Tarragon, Cilantro, Oregano, Green Onion Greens, Chives, Fennel Fronds, Thyme, Mint

Yields ~4 meals.
Accompany with toasted bread if serving as a Tapa.

Tips on how to apply

Getting Started

All you need is shrimp - everything else is flexible or a pantry staple.

Keeping it Healthy

This dish is naturally healthy - just aim for the lower end of the wide oil/butter range, adjusting to match your flavor goals. Lean protein, quick cooking, and vibrant accents make this a go-to for clean eating.

Pairings & Balance

Shrimp pairs well with a wide range of flavors - so whether you're aiming for something bright, herbaceous, spicy, or savory, the key is to keep the overall balance in mind. Let the shrimp shine, then build complementary notes around it.

Meal Prep Ideas

Shrimp works especially well in: Spring Roll, Salad, Hawaiian Protein Bowl, Soba Salad, Breakfast Burrito, Avocado Toast.

Other Tips

- Meal Prep Basic: The simplest combo (shrimp, olive oil, garlic, citrus zest and juice) makes a flexible foundation to support other dishes - layer in additional seasonings as desired for specific meals.
- Shells: Save shrimp shells for a quick, flavorful stock - just boil with salt and spices.
- Reheating: Shrimp can be enjoyed cold (especially in grain bowls or salads); if reheating, do so gently in a pan or microwave at half power to avoid toughness.
- Grilling: Grilling adds a subtle smokiness that enriches shrimp - especially with shells left on.
    - Baste with oil or marinade during grilling to add flavor and prevent sticking.

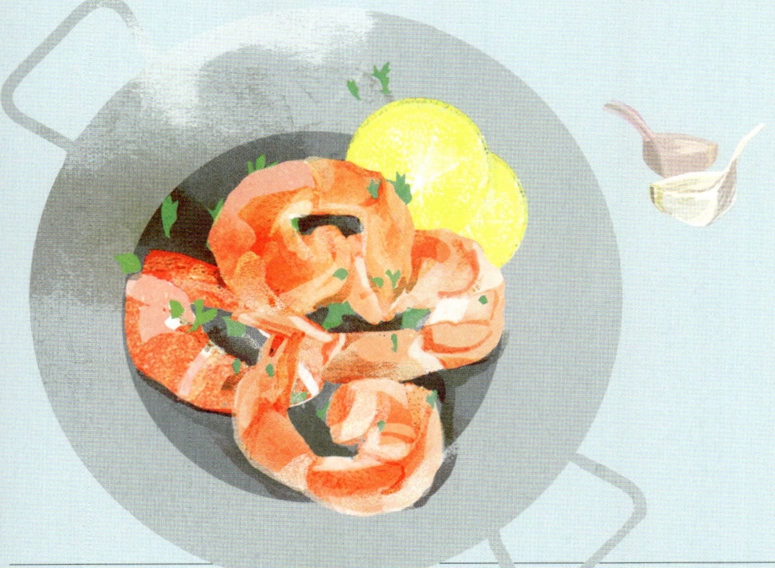

Example pairings

Meal Prep Basic

Olive Oil, Garlic, Lemon Zest + Juice

Lime Shrimp Tapa

Olive Oil, Garlic, Sherry, Lime Zest + Juice

Garnish: Parsley

Serve with: Toasted Bread

Gambas al Ajillo

Olive Oil (generous amount), Garlic (20 cloves), Paprika, Sherry, Lemon Zest + Juice; optional: Red Pepper Flakes

Garnish: Parsley

Serve with: Toasted Bread

Fra Diavolo

Olive Oil, Shallot, Garlic, Diced Tomato, Tomato Paste, Red Pepper Flakes (heavy), Calabrian Chili, White Wine, Lemon Zest + Juice

Garnish: Basil

Serve with: Linguini or similar pasta

Provençal Fennel

Butter (4-8T), Garlic, Shallot, Fennel (Bulb and/or Seed), Pastis

Garnish: Parsley +/- Fennel Frond

Serve with: Toasted Baguette

Cajun Spiced

6-12T Butter + Olive Oil, Garlic, Onion, Oregano, Cayenne, Paprika, Lemon Juice

Garnish: Parsley

Serve with: Toasted Bread

Garlic Ginger

Neutral Oil, Garlic, Ginger, Green Onion Whites, Five-Spice, Lime Zest + Juice

Garnish: Sesame Oil, Green Onion Greens +/- Cilantro

Foundational Tofu Framework

Infuse bold flavors into Tofu – whether seared, marinated or roasted.

Start by choosing whether to bake, broil, or sauté the tofu – then season or marinate accordingly to build flavor before cooking. From there, layer on sauces, herbs, acid, or garnishes to shape the final dish. Tofu absorbs what surrounds it, making it a perfect canvas for bold, expressive combinations.

Prep

1. Tofu: Select 2 lb firm or extra firm

- Cut into ~3/4″ Cubes or slice into ~1/2″ Sheets
- Blanch ~3 min in salted water or press to remove excess moisture

2. Season with Salt, plus any desired Spices

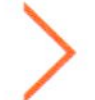

Cook

3a. Sauté

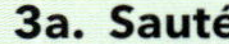

- Heat 1-3T Neutral Oil in pan on medium-high
- Add Garlic, Ginger, and/or Onion

  Veggies [optional]: Add, sequencing by hardness; push from center

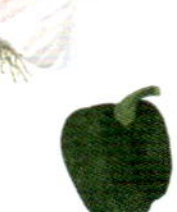

- Add Cubed Tofu, sauté ~5 min, stir occasionally, until lightly browned

  Deglaze [optional]: with 3-5T Sake, Sherry, Mirin, Wine or Stock

- Sauce: Stir in 5-10T any desired combo

OR

3b. Broil:

- Preheat Broiler, spread Tofu on baking sheet, cook ~20 min, until golden-brown

  Veggies [optional]: Lightly toss with Oil, Salt and any desired Spices

- Sauce: Brush with 4-8T, halfway through broiling

OR

3c. Bake:

- Preheat oven to 360°F (182°C)
- Add 4-8T Sauces to Tofu, bake ~50 min, until golden

  Veggies [optional]: Lightly toss with Oil, Salt and any desired Spices; add halfway through baking Tofu

Finish

4. Garnish as desired with:

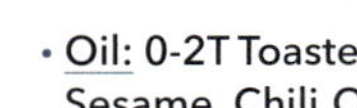

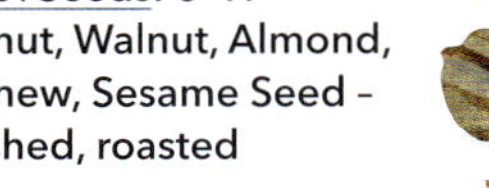

- Herbs: Fresh – chopped
- Acid: 0-2T
- Nuts /Seeds: 0-4T Peanut, Walnut, Almond, Cashew, Sesame Seed – crushed, roasted
- Oil: 0-2T Toasted Sesame, Chili Oil

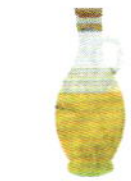

Garnish just before serving or refrigerate Tofu to add to other dishes throughout the week

Suggested Ingredients

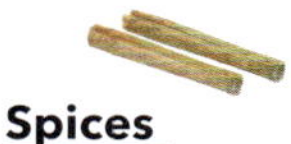

Spices

Garlic, Ginger, Miso, Peppercorn, Five-Spice, Paprika, Cumin, Coriander, Nutritional Yeast, Cayenne, Turmeric, Jerk Seasoning

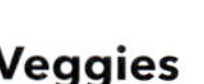

Sauces

Soy Sauce, Ponzu, Hoisin, Teriyaki, Miso, Maple Syrup, BBQ Sauce, Sesame Oil, Sriracha/Chili Paste, Pesto, Chimichurri

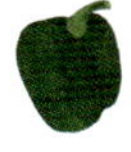

Veggies

Onion, Shiitake, Cremini, Snap Pea, Edamame, Bell Pepper, Carrot, Cabbage, Broccoli, Bok Choy, Cauliflower, Eggplant – chopped

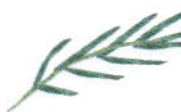

Herbs

Green Onion Greens, Cilantro, Nori, Thai Basil, Mint, Parsley, Oregano, Thyme, Dill, Sage

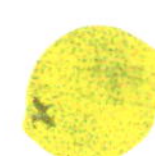

Acid:

Citrus Juice (Orange, Lime, Lemon, Yuzu) or Vinegar (Rice, Sherry, Balsamic, Cider)

Yields ~4 meals.

Tips on how to apply

Getting Started

All you need is tofu - everything else is flexible or a pantry staple.

Keeping it Healthy

Tofu is naturally healthy - just be mindful of sauces, as many contain high levels of sugar or sodium.

Pairings & Balance

Tofu is a blank canvas for whatever flavors you choose to impart. Pairing herbs, spices, and oils from the same region is a reliable way to create balanced flavors.

- Sauce: Use 2-3 sauces that offer contrast and complement each other. Combine a savory base (soy sauce, miso, BBQ) with sweet (maple, hoisin), spicy (sriracha, chili paste), or bright/herbal elements (ponzu, pesto, chimichurri).
- Sauce Quantity: Add more sauce if including lots of veggies, so everything stays well coated.

Meal Prep Ideas:

Tofu works especially well in: Quinoa Bowls, Soba Salads, Lettuce Wraps, Spring Rolls, Hawaiian Protein Bowls, Pasta Salads, Breakfast Burritos.

Other Tips

- Meal Prep Basic: The simplest combo (tofu, salt, pepper, neutral oil) makes a flexible foundation to support other dishes - layer in additional seasonings as desired for specific meals.
- Reheating: Tofu reheats easily in a pan or microwave - or enjoy cold in a Salad, Lettuce Wrap, Grain Bowl, or Sandwich.
- Grilling: Follow the same method as broiling - flip and glaze halfway through; works especially well with BBQ sauce, teriyaki, or maple syrup.
- Deep-Fry: Not included in the main framework due to added effort and lower health value - if desired: cut tofu into ~¾" cubes, pat dry thoroughly, and fry ~3 min in 2-3" of neutral, high smoke point oil until golden; drain on paper towels.

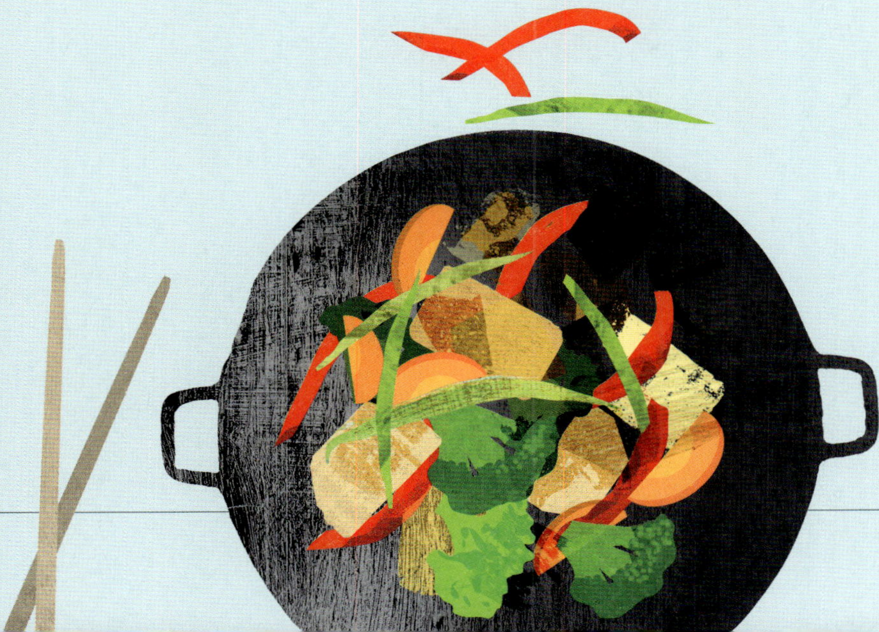

Example pairings

Sauté: Meal Prep Basic

Salt, Pepper; optional: Garlic Powder

Sauté: Neutral Oil

Sauce: Soy Sauce

Sauté: Ponzu Garlic Ginger

Sauté: Neutral Oil, Garlic, Ginger, Green Onion Whites, Mushroom, Broccoli/Bok Choy

Sauce: Mirin, Ponzu; optional: Chili Sauce

Garnish: Green Onion Greens

Sauté: Pad Thai Inspired 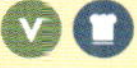

Sauté: Peanut Oil, Garlic, Ginger, Shallot, Carrot

Sauce: Soy Sauce, Ketchup, Sriracha, Brown Sugar; optional: Fish Sauce, Black Bean Sauce

Garnish: Cilantro, Peanut, Lime

Broil: Miso Glazed 

Broil: Tofu, Shiitake; optional: Carrot

Sauce: Miso Paste, Mirin, Rice Vinegar, Honey

Garnish: Green Onion, Sesame Seed

Broil/Grill: BBQ 

Grill: Neutral Oil, Tofu, Bell Pepper

Sauce: BBQ Sauce (from scratch: Ketchup, Vinegar, Sugar, Spices - simmered ~45min)

Garnish: Green Onion, additional BBQ Sauce

Bake: Maple Cajun Spiced 

Sauce: Cajun Spice Blend, Maple Syrup

Bake: Sweet Potato

Garnish: Parsley

Marinated-Roast Chicken Framework

Reinterpret this classic, with global inspiration and modern flair.

Start with a whole chicken, spatchcocked bird, or bone-in parts, then choose a dry brine or wet marinade to layer in flavor. Roast simply or build a full meal by lining the pan with seasoned veggies or fruit. Global spices, fresh herbs, and citrus variations let this classic take on new character each time.

Prep

1. Chicken: Select 3-4 lb:

- Whole: Wishbone removed for more even, faster cooking
- Spatchcocked: Backbone removed and bird flattened for faster, more even roasting
- Bone-in Parts: 8-10 pieces if from whole Chicken or equivalent cuts

2. Dry Brine or Marinate (1-24hrs in fridge):

Dry Brine: Pat dry, then, generously season all over (and under skin) with Salt & Pepper, plus optionally:

- Herbs
- Spices

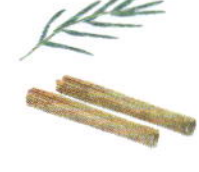

OR

Marinate: Season as above, plus:

- Oil
- Acid

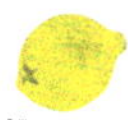

- Sweet [optional]: Honey, Sugar, Maple Syrup, Pomegranate Molasses
- Other [optional]: Greek Yogurt, Mustard, Soy Sauce, Sherry, Crushed Nuts (Almond, Cashew, Peanut)

Brine/marinate in a plastic bag or covered non-reactive bowl - the former helps ensure full coating and makes it easy to move the Chicken around

Cook

3. Prep for oven:

- Let Chicken sit at room temp 30-60 min
- Preheat oven to 425°F (218°C)
- Select large cast iron skillet, roasting pan or Dutch oven (preheat in oven for better sear)

  [optional]: Line pan with seasoned and lightly oiled Veggies and/or Fruits - sliced (peeled/cored if appropriate)

4. Roast Chicken 35-60 min, until breast internal temp reaches 165°F (74°C)

- Occasionally baste with pan juices or remaining marinade

Lower end of time range for Parts; upper end is for Whole Chicken

Finish

5. Garnish as desired with:

- Fresh Herbs
- Acid

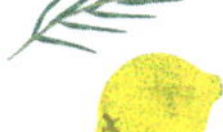

- If Carving:
- Let Chicken rest ~10 min to retain juices
- Separate the legs and thighs by slicing through the skin at the joints
- Remove wings
- Finally, slice the breasts against the grain

Suggested Ingredients

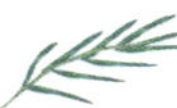
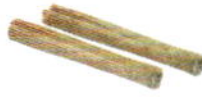
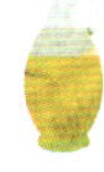
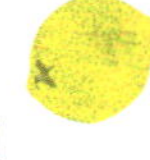
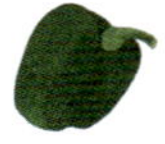

Herbs	Spices	Oil	Acid	Veggies	Fruits
Cilantro, Parsley, Rosemary, Thyme, Tarragon, Oregano, Sage	Minced Garlic, Red Pepper Flakes, Ginger, Lemongrass, Paprika, Coriander, Cumin, Cardamom, Cinnamon, Turmeric, Star Anise	Olive, Avocado, Butter, Neutral Oil	Citrus Slices and Juice (Lemon, Orange, Lime), Vinegar (White Wine, Balsamic, Rice)	Potato, Sweet Potato, Fennel, Leek, Carrot, Parsnip, Mushroom, Brussels Sprout, Kale, Celery Root, Squash	Apple, Pear, Apricot, Clementine

Serves 4.

Tips on how to apply

Getting Started

All you need is chicken and a pan big enough to roast it in - everything else is flexible or a kitchen staple.

Keeping it Healthy

This is a high-protein, balanced dish that leans healthy even with the skin on. To maximize healthiness, skip eating the skin and opt for marinades free from butter or added sugar.

Pairings & Balance

Roast on a bed of sliced veggies to let the juices infuse flavor while also rounding out the meal - see Roast Veggies framework for inspiration. Brighten richness with fresh herbs and citrus zest.

Other Tips

- Butchering: Ask your butcher to handle the prep - whether removing the wishbone, spatchcocking, or separating into parts.
- Truss: For whole chickens, tie the legs with kitchen twine and tuck in the wing tips to promote even cooking and retain moisture.
- Simple Gravy: Deglaze pan with wine or stock, whisk in 1-2t flour/ cornstarch, and simmer until thickened.
- Crispy Skin: Don't be alarmed if the skin darkens deeply - that caramelization adds flavor. For extra crispness, consider broiling during the final 5 minutes.
- Duck: For a ~5 lb duck, skip the oil - it's naturally rich in fat; score the skin to help render.
    - Brush with marinade twice during roasting.
    - Roast ~50 min for parts, ~70 min for a whole bird, until internal temp reaches 155°F (68°C).
    - Flavor Affinities: Honey, lavender, garlic, ginger, clove, orange, lemon, mushroom, sweet potato, soy sauce.

Example pairings

Classic Garlic & Herb

Dry Brine: Thyme, Rosemary, Garlic, Black Pepper

Optional Veggies: Potato, Carrot, and/or Onion

Garnish: Parsley, Lemon Wedges

Smoked Paprika & Orange

Dry Brine: Smoked Paprika, Garlic, Orange Zest, Black Pepper

Optional Veggies: Red Onion, Sweet Potato, and/or Bell Pepper

Garnish: Cilantro, Orange Slices

Middle Eastern Spiced

Dry Brine: Parsley, Garlic, Za'atar, Sumac, Cumin, Red Pepper Flakes

Optional Veggies: Red Onion, Fennel

Garnish: Parsley, Pomegranate Seed

Harissa & Lemon

Marinade: Lemon Juice, Olive Oil, Harissa Paste, Garlic, Coriander, Cumin

Optional Veggies: Sweet Potato, Carrot

Garnish: Mint, Lemon Wedges

Lemon Garlic Yogurt

Marinade: Lemon Juice, Plain Greek Yogurt, Olive Oil, Garlic, Oregano, Thyme

Optional Veggies: Tomato, Onion, and/or Zucchini

Garnish: Parsley, Lemon Wedges

Thai Coconut Lime

Marinade: Lime Juice, Coconut Oil, Ginger, Lemongrass, Chili Flakes, Fish Sauce

Optional Veggies: Green Onion, Mushroom, Baby Corn

Garnish: Thai Basil, Lime Wedges

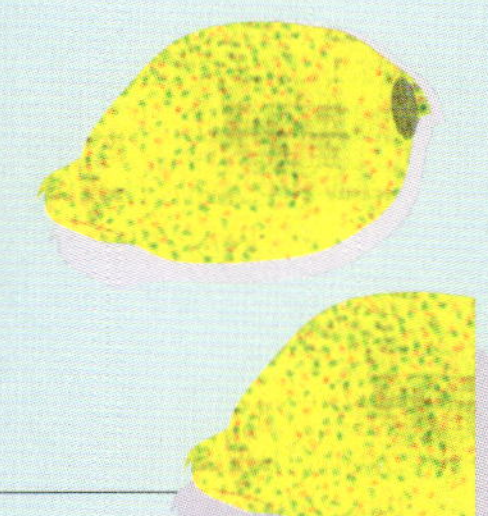

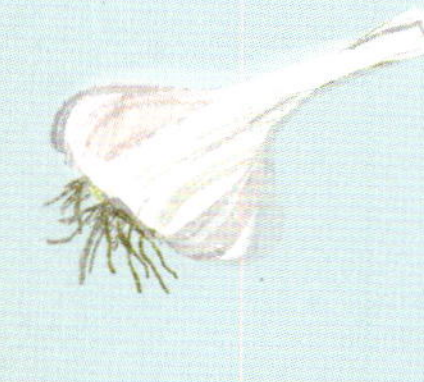

Pantry & Prep

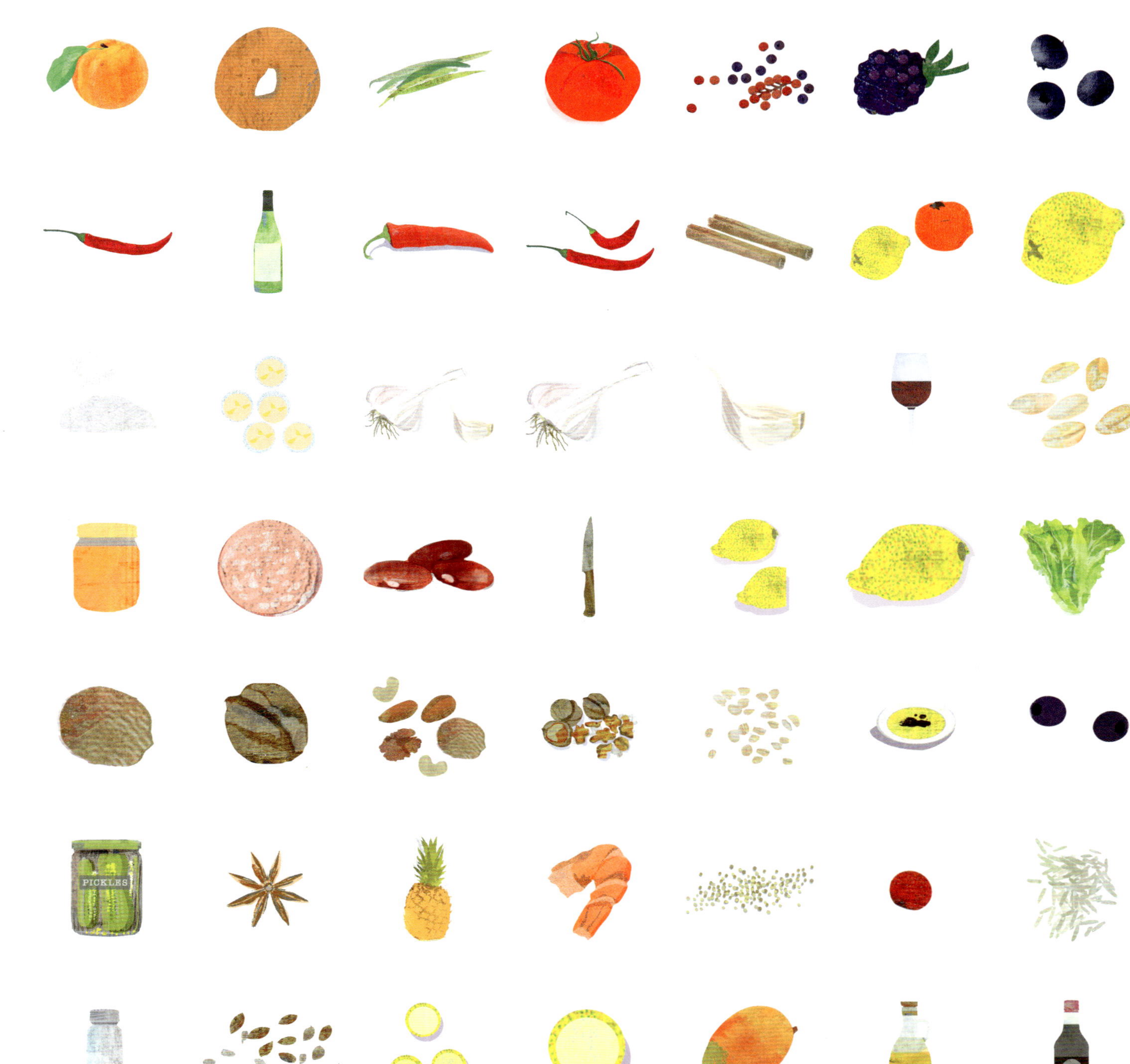

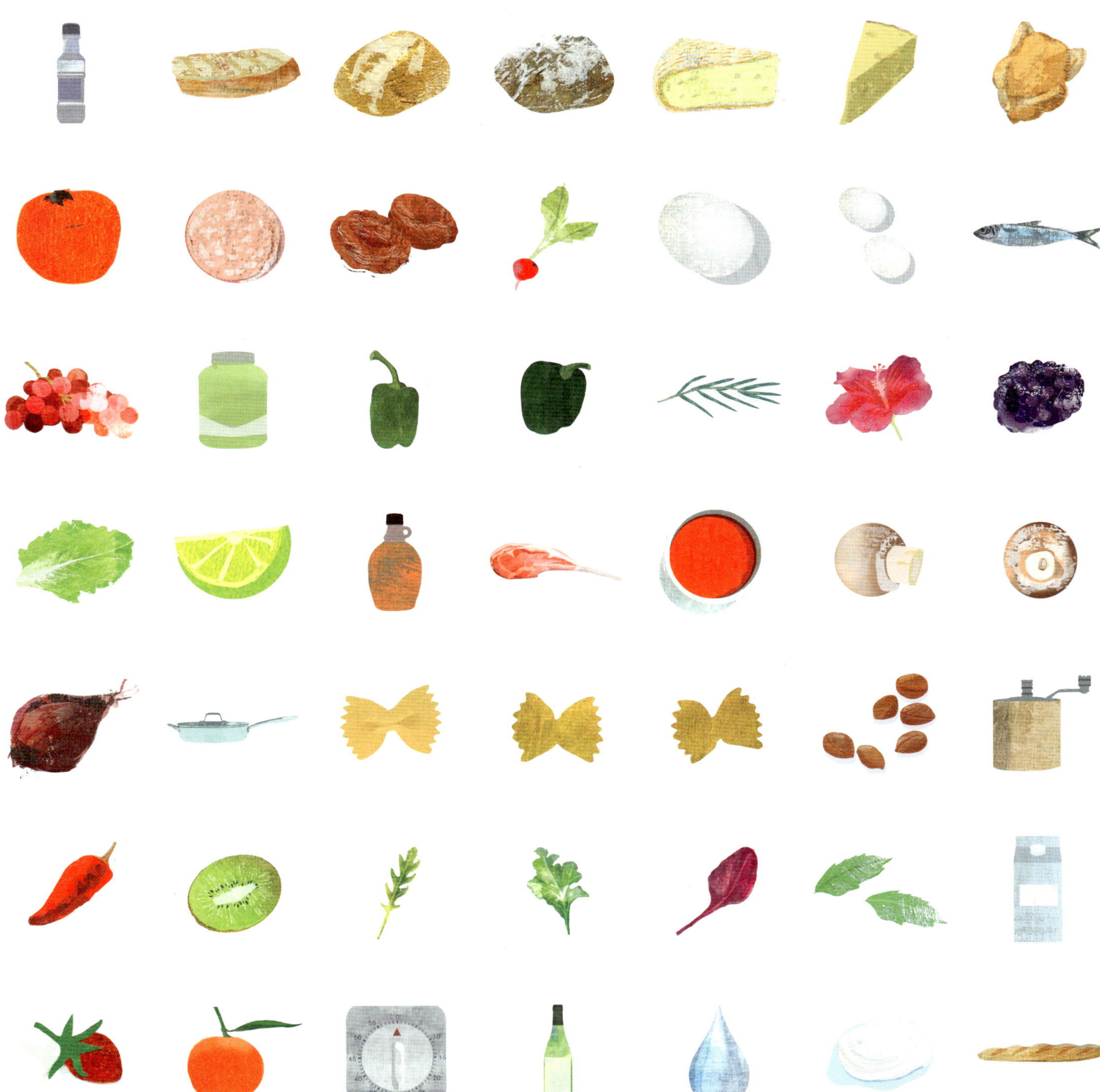

Pantry Builder

Build your pantry by selecting your favorite ingredients spanning key categories, starting with essentials and phasing in more esoteric ingredients.

Shelf Stable

Oil

- Olive
- Butter
- Avocado
- Chili
- Sesame
- Ghee
- Canola/Corn
- Grapeseed
- Truffle
- Coconut

Vinegar

- Balsamic
- White Wine
- Red Wine
- Rice-Unseasoned
- Rice-Seasoned
- Apple Cider
- Champagne
- Sherry
- Umeboshi
- Chinkiang

Seasonings

- Salt-Kosher
- Salt-Sea/Fleur de Sel
- Salt-Himalayan Pink
- Black Pepper
- Red Pepper Flakes
- Cayenne
- White Pepper
- Sichuan/Mala Pepper
- Cinnamon
- Coriander
- Cumin
- Paprika
- Garlic Powder
- Ginger Powder
- Vanilla Bean/Extract
- Cardamom
- Clove
- Nutmeg
- Sesame Seed
- Turmeric
- Allspice
- Fennel Seed
- Five-Spice
- Garam Masala
- Gochugaru
- Mustard Seed
- Nutritional Yeast
- Onion Powder
- Ras-el-Hanout
- Star Anise
- Sumac
- Togarashi
- Wasabi
- Celery Seed
- Galangal Powder
- Mace
- Za'atar

Herbs

- Basil*
- Cilantro*
- Mint*
- Oregano
- Parsley*
- Rosemary
- Tarragon*
- Thyme
- Bay Leaf
- Herbes de Provence
- Chives
- Dill
- Kaffir Lime Leaf
- Lavender
- Lemongrass
- Nori
- Orange Peel
- Saffron
- Sage
- Shiso
- Chervil
- Marjoram
- Savory

**Particularly preferable fresh – having dried provides a helpful base for improvisation*

Stock

- Chicken
- Vegetable
- Beef
- Seafood
- Fish

Grains

- Rice-White
- Rice-Jasmine
- Rice-Brown
- Rice-Arborio
- Rice-Calasparra
- Pasta-Penne/Bow Tie
- Pasta-Spaghetti
- Pasta-Lasagna
- Soba Noodle
- Udon Noodle
- Quinoa
- Vermicelli
- Barley/Faro
- Couscous
- Dumpling Wrapper
- Rolled Oats
- Spring Roll Wrapper

Sweeteners

- Sugar-White
- Sugar-Brown
- Honey
- Maple Syrup
- Agave Syrup
- Coconut/Palm Sugar

Baking Essentials

- Baking Soda
- Flour
- Breadcrumb/Panko
- Cornstarch
- Baking Powder
- Cocoa Powder
- Yeast

Chili Sauce

- Chili Crisp
- Hot Sauce
- Harissa/Sambal
- Sriracha
- Gochujang
- Sweet Chili Sauce

Sauce

- Tomato Paste
- Mustard
- Soy Sauce
- Mayo
- Miso
- Ponzu
- Sherry
- Tahini
- Tomato Sauce
- Coconut Milk
- Fish Sauce
- Hoisin
- Ketchup
- Mirin
- Shaoxing Wine
- Oyster Sauce
- Pesto
- Yuzu Paste
- Shrimp Paste

Supplements

- Protein Powder
- Chia Seed
- Flax Seed
- Green Powder
- Creatine

Essential
Valuable
Useful
Specialized
Niche

Prioritization reflects the usefulness of keeping an item stocked for cooking the dishes in this book – longer shelf life means more opportunities to use it.

This list is light on fresh items, as they're best bought with intention. Still, a few – like bell pepper, tomato, and lemon – are so versatile they're often worth keeping on hand.

Nuts/Seeds

- Peanut
- Almond
- Cashew
- Pistachio
- Walnut
- Macadamia
- Pepita/Pumpkin Seed
- Sunflower Seed
- Hazelnut
- Pecan

Beans

- Chickpea
- Lentil
- Black Bean
- Cannellini/White

Dried Fruit

- Apricot
- Prune
- Raisin
- Apple
- Coconut Flake
- Date
- Fig
- Lemon/Lime Wheel
- Mango

Dried Veg

- Chili-Ancho/Chipotle
- Chili-Sichuan
- Shiitake
- Porcini
- Fried Shallot
- Morel

Frozen

Frozen Veggie

- Edamame
- Corn
- Peas
- Broccoli
- Spinach
- Carrot
- Green Beans
- Mixed Veggie

Frozen Fruit

- Banana
- Blueberry
- Pineapple
- Strawberry
- Açaí
- Mango
- Peach
- Mixed Berry
- Avocado
- Blackberry
- Raspberry
- Aloe
- Cherry
- Dragon Fruit
- Jackfruit
- Papaya

Frozen Protein

- Chicken Breast
- Fish
- Shrimp
- Bison Burger
- Tempeh
- Veggie Burger

Semi-Perishable

Jarred Veg/Fruit

- Olive
- Sun-dried Tomato
- Artichoke
- Calabrian Chili
- Caper
- Pickled Cucumber
- Diced Tomato
- Jalapeño
- Pickled Onion
- Roasted Pepper
- Banana Pepper
- Cornichon
- Garlic
- Giardiniera
- Kimchi
- Bamboo Shoot
- Pickled Beet
- Pickled Carrot/Corn
- Heart of Palm
- Pickled Ginger
- Preserved Lemon
- Straw Mushroom

Cured Meat

- Spanish Chorizo
- Prosciutto
- Salami/Pepperoni
- Anchovy
- Bacon
- Deli Ham
- Deli Beef
- Deli Chicken

Roots

- Garlic
- Onion-Yellow
- Onion-Red
- Onion-White
- Ginger
- Shallot
- Potato
- Sweet Potato
- Jicama

Dairy & Egg

- Egg
- Parmesan
- Feta
- Mozzarella
- Ricotta
- Burrata
- Cottage Cheese
- Pecorino
- Queso Fresco
- Provolone
- Cream Cheese
- Mascarpone
- Yogurt-Greek
- Yogurt-Plain
- Yogurt-Vanilla
- Milk/Substitute
- Cream
- Crème Fraîche
- Sour Cream
- Buttermilk

Perishable

Fresh Veggie

- Bell Pepper
- Green Onion
- Mushroom-Cremini
- Tomato
- Arugula
- Avocado
- Carrot
- Lettuce
- Cucumber

Fresh Fruit

- Lemon
- Lime
- Banana
- Orange
- Apple
- Pear
- Blueberry
- Grapefruit
- Strawberry
- Peach/Nectarine
- Pineapple

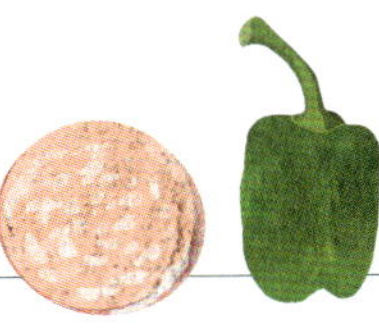

Internal Temperature & Doneness Guide

Key

- ● Chef Recommended
- ◆ USDA Min

Temperature

°F	100	110	120	130	140	150	160	170	180	190	200
°C	38	43	49	54	60	66	71	77	82	88	93

	Item	Chef Recommended (°F / °C)	USDA Min (°F / °C)	Doneness Cues
Beef	**Lean Steaks** (Filet Mignon, Loin, Sirloin, Flank)	*Medium-Rare* 130 / 54	145 / 63	Slightly firm edges; red-pink center
	Fatty Steaks Rib Eye, Chuck Eye	*Medium* 135 / 54	145 / 63	Fat rendered; pink center
	Braising Cuts Chuck, Brisket, Short Rib	>180 / >82	145 / 63	Fork-tender; easily pulls apart
	Ground	160 / 71	160 / 71	Browned; no pink
Poultry	**Chicken White Meat** Breast	155 / 68	165 / 74	Firm; opaque; juices clear
	Chicken Dark Meat Thigh, Drumstick	160 / 71	165 / 74	Tender, easily pulls from bone
	Ground Poultry Chicken, Turkey	165 / 74	165 / 74	No pink
Pork	**Lean Cuts** (Chop, Loin, Tenderloin)	*Medium-Rare* 145 / 63	145 / 63	Slight blush pink
	Braising Cuts (Shoulder, Belly)	>180 / >82	145 / 63	Fork-tender; easily shredded
	Ground	160 / 71	160 / 71	Browned; no pink
Lamb	**Tender Cuts** (Chops, Loin, Leg)	*Rare to Medium-Rare* 130-135 / 54-57	145 / 63	Rosy pink center
	Braising Cuts (Shoulder, Shank, Bone-in Leg)	>180 / >82	145 / 63	Fork-tender; easily pulls apart
	Ground	160 / 71	160 / 71	Browned; no pink
Seafood	**Tuna** (Seared Ahi)	*Rare* 105-115 / 41-46	145 / 63	Brown sear; red center
	Salmon	*Medium-Rare* 120-125 / 49-52	145 / 63	Opaque outside; translucent center
	Whole Fish (Branzino, Snapper, Cod, Haddock)	135-140 / 57-60	145 / 63	Flesh opaque; flakes easily
	Shrimp	125-135 / 52-57	145 / 63	Opaque pink; curled to "C"
	Scallop	115 / 46	145 / 63	Opaque milky white
Eggs	**Eggs**	160 / 71	160 / 71	Whites set; yolks runny to firm
Leftovers	**Leftovers**	165 / 74	165 / 74	Steaming hot throughout

Disclaimer: To minimize risk of foodborne illness, follow USDA guidelines for minimum internal temperatures – especially for vulnerable populations. When in doubt, heat to 165°F (74°C).

Source: USDA Minimums: https://www.fsis.usda.gov/food-safety/safe-food-handling-and-preparation/food-safety-basics/safe-temperature-chart

Oils by Flavor, Smoke Point, and Healthiness

Select the optimal oil based on smoke point, flavor, and overall health profile.

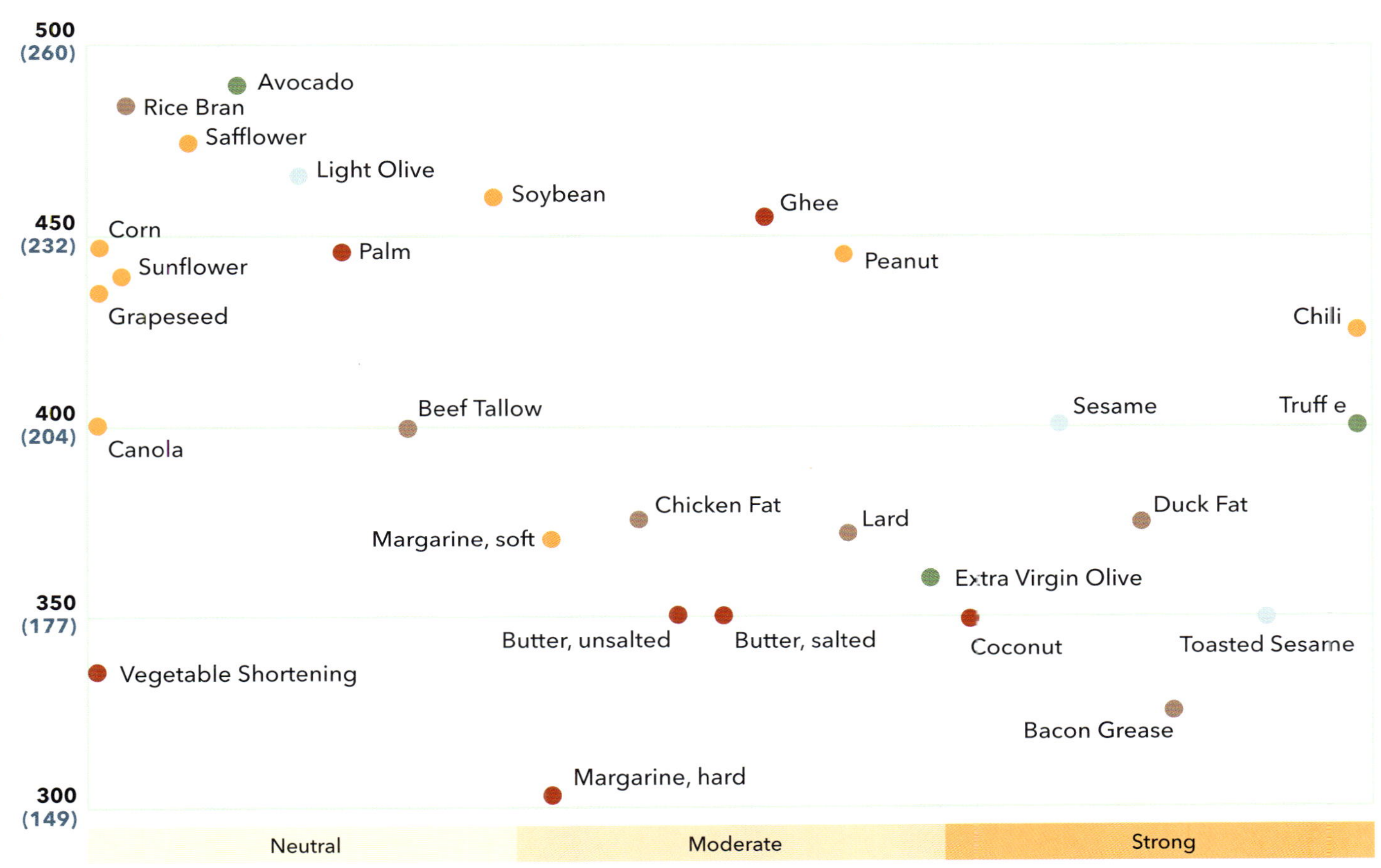

Flavor Strength

Key

- Nutrient-Dense Oils: High in Omega-3 and/or considered anti-inflammatory
- Neither associated with significant health benefits nor concerns
- Refined Seed Oils with <25% Saturated Fat: Lower in saturated fat, though some raise concerns due to industrial extraction methods
- Moderate Saturated Fat (25-50%)
- High Trans/Saturated Fat (>50%)

Smoke points may vary by refinement and environmental factors. Vegetable oil not included as it can be a varying mix of refined seed oils.

CookImprov Core Oils

Go-To

Extra Virgin Olive Oil: Flavor-forward; great for general cooking and dressings

Avocado Oil: Neutral flavor; ideal for high-heat applications

Accents

Toasted Sesame Oil: Adds rich, nutty depth; best as a finishing oil

Chili Oil: Brings heat and punch; ideal as a finishing drizzle or in a sauce

Butter: Adds classic flavor; try cutting with olive oil

Ghee: For Indian dishes; higher smoke point than butter

Glossary & Herb/Spice Blends

Perfect your own Herb/Spice blends or whip up a quick substitute if there's one you're missing.

Herb/Spice blend ingredients are listed in order of suggested quantities. Adjust to taste and don't worry about having every ingredient – even just a few can get you most of the way there.

Improvise freely – use more of what you love, tweak, adjust, and you'll create a superior custom blend.

Advieh: Cinnamon, Cardamom, Rose Petal/Bud, Ginger, Turmeric, Cumin, Clove, Coriander

Baharat: Paprika, Peppercorn, Cumin, Cinnamon, Nutmeg, Clove, Coriander, Allspice, Turmeric

Berbere: Chili Powder*, Paprika, Garlic, Ginger, (Holy) Basil, Coriander, Fenugreek, Cardamom

Bouquet Garni: Thyme, Parsley, Bay Leaf (tied with a string/cheesecloth to easily remove from stews once cooked)

Cajun Seasoning: Paprika, Garlic Powder, Onion Powder, Cayenne, Peppercorn, Oregano, Thyme

Chermoula: Dry: Garlic (Powder), Cumin, Coriander, Parsley, Peppercorn, Paprika; Wet: Add Olive Oil, Lemon Juice

Chia Seeds: Supplement to add protein, fiber, and nutrients with little taste impact; absorbs water to form a gel-like consistency

Chimichurri: Parsley, Olive Oil, Wine Vinegar, Garlic, Oregano, Red Pepper Flakes, Salt

Clams: To clean: scrub shells then soak in 6c cold water with 3T dissolved (sea) salt for 2-4 hours so clams purge their sand/gunk

Commercial spice blends often include salt, which is excluded here as dishes will be salted separately.

Creole Seasoning: Paprika, (Celery) Salt, Oregano, Thyme, Basil, Garlic Powder, Onion Powder, Peppercorn, Cayenne, Bay Leaf, Coriander

Daikon: Large, mild-flavored white radish; eaten raw in salads, pickled, or cooked in soups/stir fries

Dukkah: Hazelnut, Sesame Seed, Coriander, Cumin, Fennel Seed, Cayenne

Fines Herbes: Parsley, Chives, Tarragon, Chervil

Five-Spice: Cinnamon, Anise Seed, Ginger Powder, Clove, Fennel Seed

Flax Seeds: Supplement to add fiber and omega-3's; often added to smoothies, oatmeal, or baked goods

Furikake: Sesame Seed, Nori, Salt, Sugar, Red Pepper Flakes, Bonito, Shiso

Galangal: Ginger-like spicy root, commonly used in Thai and other Southeast Asian cuisine

Garam Masala: Cumin, Coriander, Peppercorn, Cinnamon, Cardamom, Ginger Powder, Red Pepper Flakes, Nutmeg, Allspice, Clove, Mace, Bay Leaf, Fenugreek, Star Anise, Caraway

Ghee: Clarified butter most used in Indian cuisine – to make: simmer butter in pan on low heat, cook 15-25 min until more translucent (hence, clarified); strain; chill

Gochujang: Korean fermented Chili Paste

Gremolata: Italian Condiment of Parsley, Lemon Zest, Garlic, Salt; optional: Olive Oil, Pepper

Harissa: Chili Paste** with Olive Oil, Garlic, Coriander, Cumin, Caraway; optional: Lemon Juice

Herbes de Provence: Lavender, Rosemary, Thyme, Parsley, Tarragon, Marjoram/Oregano, Basil, Sage, Savory, Chervil

Italian Seasoning: Oregano, Basil, Thyme, Rosemary, Garlic Powder, Onion Powder, Parsley, Marjoram, Sage, Savory

Jerk Seasoning: Allspice, Garlic Powder, Cayenne, Red Pepper Flakes, Thyme, Sugar, Cinnamon, Clove, Nutmeg, Peppercorn, Paprika; optional: Onion Powder

Jicama: Slightly sweet root vegetable with a water chestnut-like texture; commonly eaten raw in salads, spring rolls, or as a crunchy snack

Kohlrabi: Crunchy vegetable tasting between cabbage and broccoli; peeled, then often eaten raw or roasted

Lardons: Small cubes of fatty bacon/pork belly

Lotus Root: Crunchy, starchy vegetable with slightly sweet flavor, often pickled, stir-fried, or added to soup

Marsala Wine: Italian cooking wine, can be dry or sweet; substitute: other cooking wine or wine; note: not to be confused with Garam Masala

Mirin: Japanese sweet cooking wine; substitute: other cooking wine/sake/ white wine + pinch of sugar

Mulling Spices: Cinnamon, Clove, Allspice, Nutmeg, Star Anise, Orange Peel

Mussels: To clean: rinse then soak in 6c cold water with 2T dissolved (sea) salt for 20–60 min; scrub and debeard just before cooking to maximize freshness

Nori: Roasted seaweed used for sushi and as a garnish

Nutritional Yeast: Vegan cheese-substitute, high protein, low fat – use as garnish similar to Parmesan

Old Bay Seasoning: Celery Salt, Paprika, Peppercorn, Mustard, Bay Leaf, Cinnamon, Clove, Nutmeg, Ginger

Parsnip: Pale carrot-like root vegetable with a sweeter, nuttier flavor; often roasted, mashed, or stewed

Pickling Spice: Coriander, Allspice, Mustard Seed, Cinnamon, Bay Leaf, Ginger Powder, Red Pepper Flakes, Clove, Peppercorn, Cardamom, Mace, Dill

Pilpelchuma: Chili Paste** with Garlic, Olive Oil, Lemon Juice, Cumin, Caraway

Ponzu: 45% Soy Sauce, 45% Vinegar/ Citrus Juice, 10% Mirin

Quatre Épices: Peppercorn, Nutmeg, Clove, Ginger Powder (or Cinnamon)

Poultry Seasoning: Sage, Thyme, Marjoram/Oregano, Rosemary, Peppercorn, Garlic, Onion Powder, Ginger, Nutmeg, Paprika

Pumpkin Spice: Cinnamon, Nutmeg, Ginger Powder, Clove, Allspice

Ras-el-Hanout: Cumin, Coriander, Cinnamon, Ginger Powder, Paprika, Peppercorn, Turmeric, Allspice, Clove, Cardamom and Nutmeg

Roux: Thickening agent made by gradually adding flour to oil/butter in pan on low heat while constantly stirring; use as base for sauce/ soup/stew

Sambal: Chili Sauce** with Garlic, Ginger, Shallot, Lime Juice, Sugar, Shrimp Paste

Sriracha/Tương Ớt: Chili Sauce** with Vinegar, Garlic, Sugar

Shaoxing Wine: Chinese dry cooking wine; substitute: dry sherry, sake, other cooking wine, or Mirin (reduce sugar slightly to balance Mirin's sweetness)

Shiso: Herb similar to Perilla, with a flavor that's a mix of mint, basil, and spice, often used in sushi and salads

Soba: Thin buckwheat-based noodles, often served chilled with dipping sauce or in broths

Soda: aka Soda Water – simply carbonated water – no sugar or quinine added

Taro: Starchy root vegetable with a slightly sweet, nutty flavor, used in savory and sweet dishes

Togarashi: Chili Powder*, Sesame Seed, Red Pepper Flakes, Orange Peel, White Pepper, Nori, Ginger Powder, Salt

Veggies: Informal term for vegetables – given its informality, the category contains items that are colloquially, if not technically, vegetables (e.g., tomatoes, cucumbers, squash, mushrooms)

Yuca/Cassava: Starchy tuber, often used in Latin American and African cuisine, served boiled or fried

Yuzu Kosho: Condiment fermented from combination of Yuzu Zest, Green Chili, and Salt

Za'atar (blend): Thyme, Sumac, Sesame Seed, Za'atar (herb)

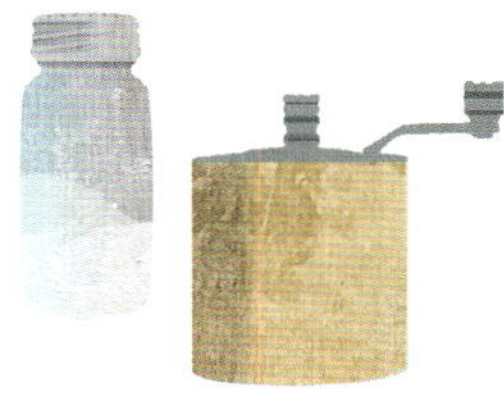

Key	Spice Blend	Blend w/ Chili Powder	Blend with Chili Paste or Chili Sauce
	To Make:	***Chili Powder**: Grind, blend, or finely chop dried chilis – with or without their seeds.	**Chili Paste/Sauce: Steam, boil, or roast a mix of mild and hot peppers then blend – seeds optional. Adjust liquid for a thinner sauce or thicker paste. Quick substitute: dice marinated Calabrian Chili or use Red Pepper Flakes, instead of fresh chili/pepper.

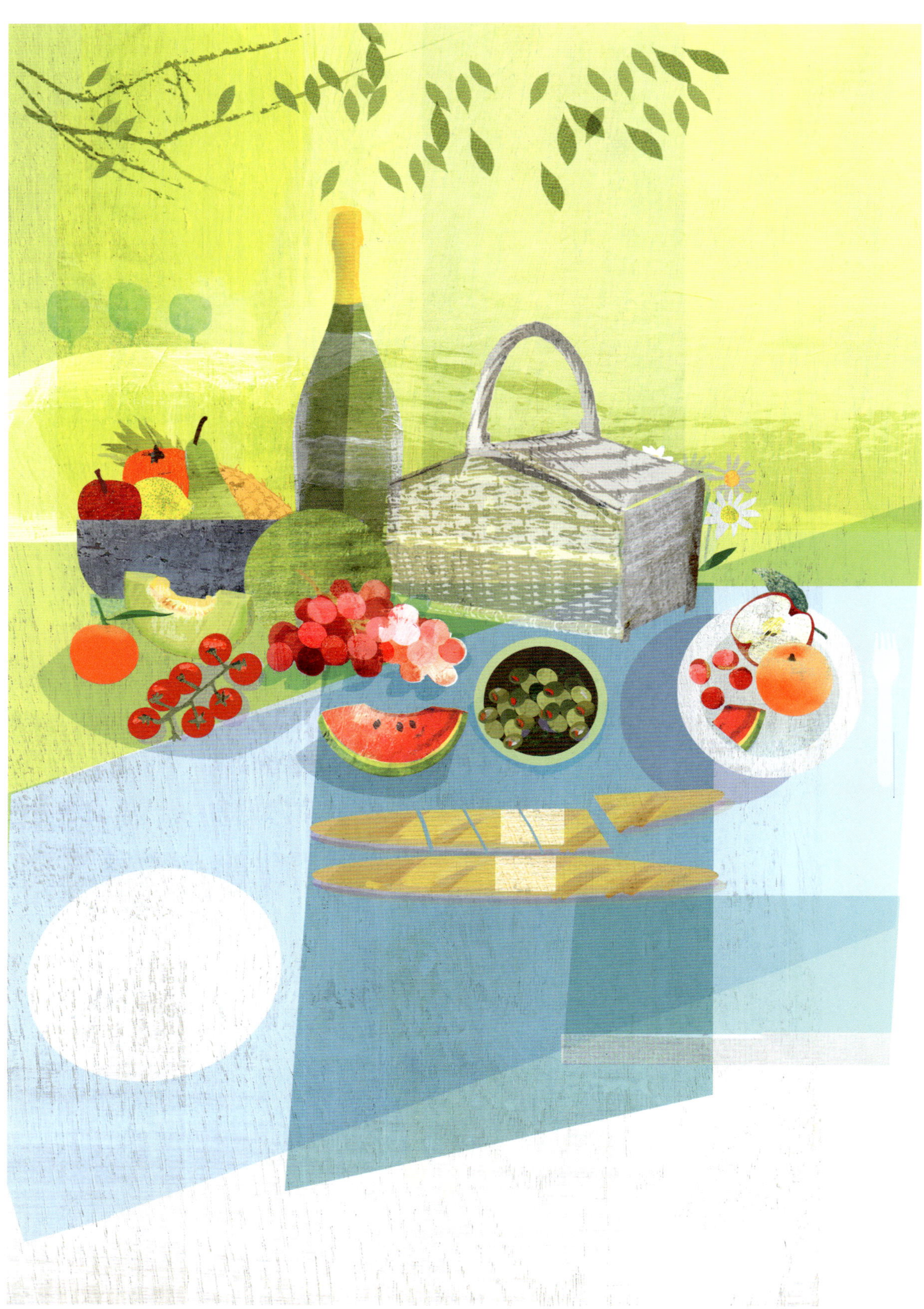

Reflections

I hope your experience with this book has been a liberating journey, and along the way, you've crafted a dish that became a favorite and is uniquely yours.

Food is one of the most universal forms of connection - it brings people together, sparks conversation, and deepens appreciation for different cultures. Every cuisine tells a story, shaped by tradition, geography, and generations of humans improvising with what's available. When we cook, we're not just feeding ourselves - we're engaging in an art form that fosters understanding, generosity, and creativity.

Beyond the kitchen, creativity fuels fulfillment. Whether you're experimenting with flavors or brainstorming new ideas, the ability to build, adapt, and refine drives progress. The same "yes, and" mindset that makes improvisational cooking so freeing applies just as well to everyday problem-solving, personal projects, and professional challenges.

Whether crafting a dish, designing a project, or simply thinking through a challenge, continue to improvise, iterate, and create with confidence, curiosity, and an openness to experiment.

Thank You!

This book exists thanks to the support, encouragement, and talents of so many extraordinary people. To my family, friends, creative collaborators, and the publishing team – thank you for believing in my vision and helping bring it to life.

To my Mother and Nonna, who taught me how to cook – and to memories of chaotic brilliance with Jillian Barber, who said "yes, and" to flambéing an alligator in our college dorm.

To the friends who offered encouragement, perspective, and support along the way: Jon Chan, David Chiu, Hoshang Chenoy, Hans Gildenhuys, Whitney Hallock, Christian Jensen, Diana Kim, Jacob Kim, Vincent Ko, Larry Luchtel, Tanay Nagpal, Isaac Olvera, Peter Peterson, Jeremy Svenson, Rebecca Raybin, Robin Respaut, Michael Tsai, Sean Water, Darlene Yang, Yang Yang, and Kenichi Young – thank you for the energy and conviction when I needed it most.

I'm profoundly grateful to Lou Baker Smith, the luminous illustrator who captured the spirit of CookImprov; to Kat Catmur, the visionary art director who composed its visual rhythm, giving structure to its spontaneity; to Karen Constanti, the magnificent designer whose craft gave each spread balance and beauty; and to Judith Doyle, the meticulous editor whose sharp eye refined every line. Deep thanks also to my wise and candid advisors, Vanessa Poster and MeiMei Fox, for their insights throughout the journey.

To my partner, Hoon Bae: thanks for your endless support, discerning palate, and for rigorously testing these frameworks with care, humor, and love.

And to you, my readers – thank you for joining me on this journey. I hope this book continues to spark your creativity and inspire you to create dishes that surpass my own.

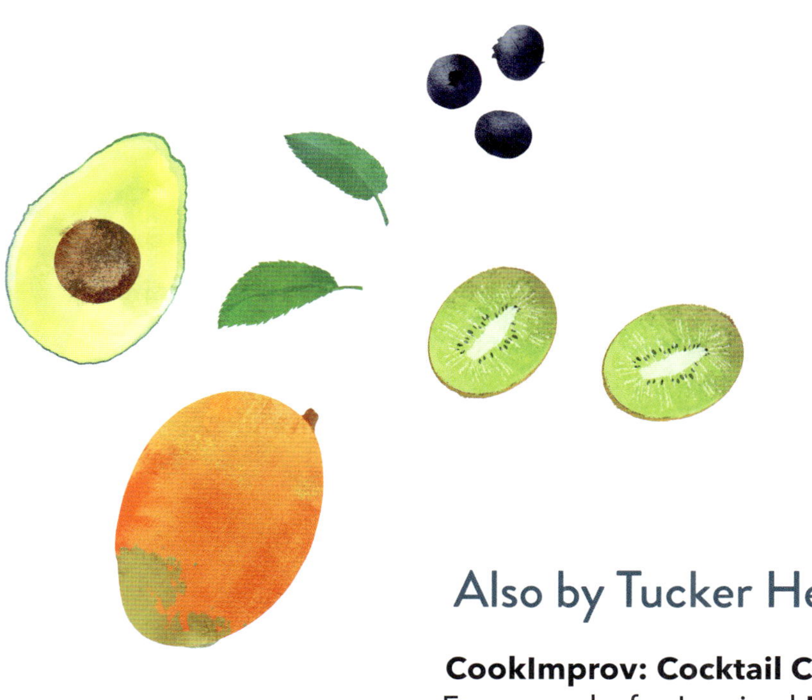

Also by Tucker Herbert

CookImprov: Cocktail Creations
Frameworks for Inspired Mixology

(coming early 2026)

CookImprov: Masterpiece Methods
Frameworks for Signature Dishes,
Global Flavors, and Techniques

(coming late 2026)

Connect with the CookImprov Community

www.cookimprov.com

Instagram: @cookimprov
TikTok: @cookimprov
YouTube: @cookimprov

Share your creations,
get inspired, and keep improvising.

Notes

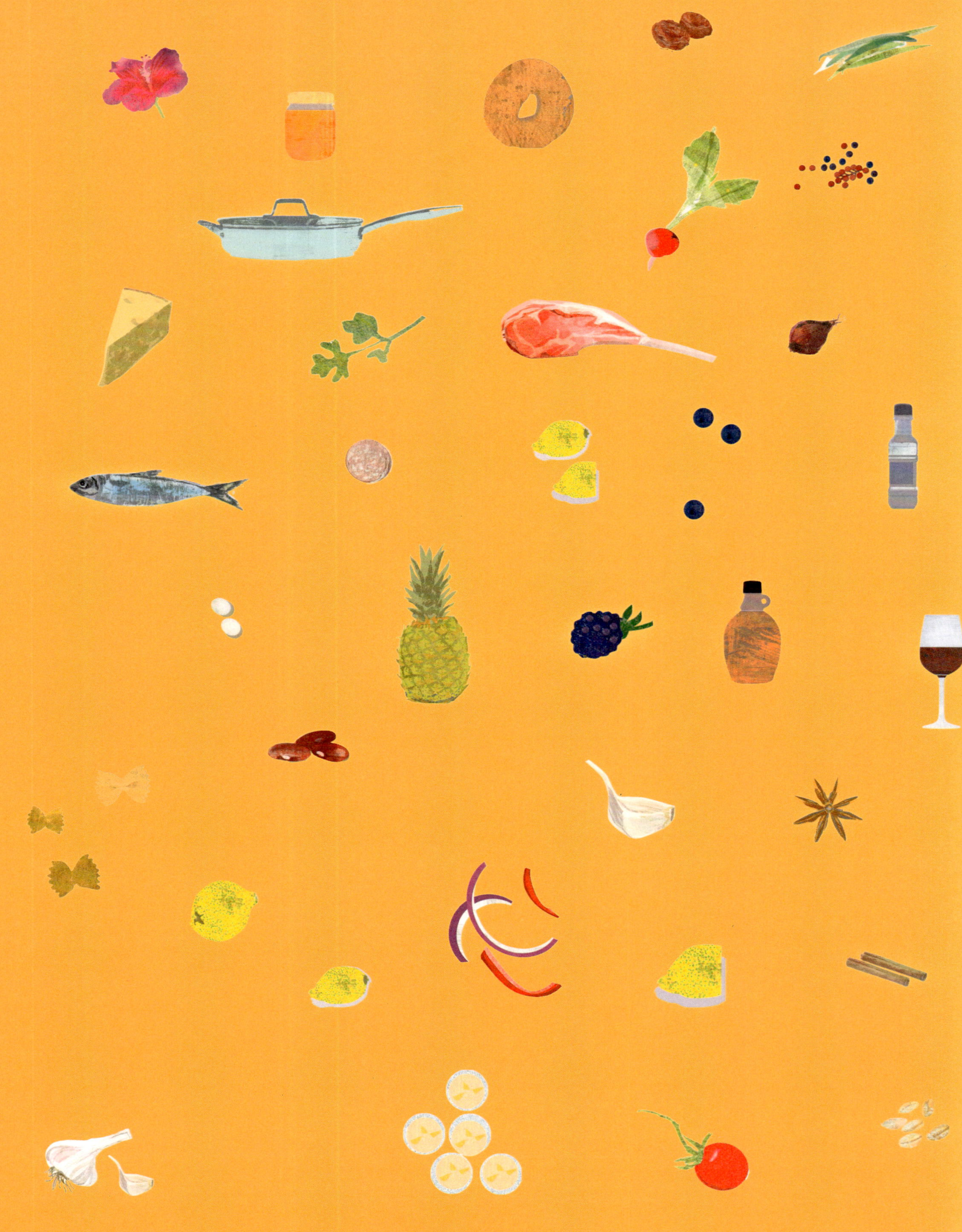